Outwit your Weight

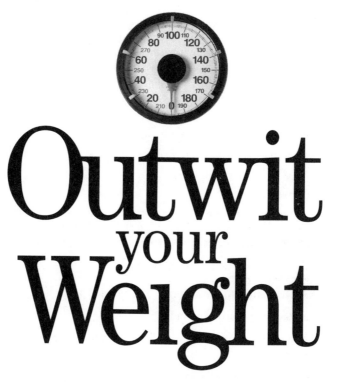

Outwit your Weight

FAT-PROOF YOUR LIFE WITH MORE THAN 200 TIPS, TOOLS, & TECHNIQUES TO HELP YOU DEFEAT YOUR DIET DANGER ZONES

By CATHY NONAS, R.D.

Director, VanItallie Center for Nutrition and Weight Management at St. Luke's–Roosevelt Hospital

with Julia VanTine

RODALE

© 2002 by Cathy Nonas

Printed in the United States of America
Rodale Inc. makes every effort to use acid-free ∞, recycled paper ♻.

Cover and interior design by Carol Angstadt

Photographs by Andrew Cameron (pen), EyeWire Collection (scale), and Hilmar (Cathy Nonas)

Library of Congress Cataloging-in-Publication Data

Nonas, Cathy.
   Outwit your weight : fat-proof your life with more than 200 tips, tools, and techniques to help you defeat your diet danger zones / by Cathy Nonas, with Julia VanTine.
       p.   cm.
   Includes index.
   ISBN 1–57954–482–7   hardcover
   1. Weight loss.   I. VanTine, Julia.   II. Title.
RM222.2 .N655   2002
613.2'5—dc21   2001007027

Distributed to the book trade by St. Martin's Press

2   4   6   8   10   9   7   5   3   1   hardcover

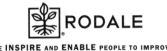

RODALE

WE INSPIRE AND ENABLE PEOPLE TO IMPROVE THEIR LIVES AND THE WORLD AROUND THEM

FOR MORE OF OUR PRODUCTS
WWW.RODALESTORE.COM
(800) 848-4735

To the men and women in my Wednesday
night and Thursday morning classes. You inspire me.
To Aurora, Sasha, and Lucy, who eat smart, and are.
—*Cathy Nonas*

To my beautiful son, Wyeth Daniel.
May you live, always, in health, happiness, and peace.
—*Julia VanTine*

Contents

Acknowledgments

So many people encouraged me to write this book. First, I'd like to thank Xavier Pi-Sunyer, M.D., and Theodore B. VanItallie, M.D., both of whom trusted me to put into practice everything they taught me.

I'd also like to thank the staff of the VanItallie Center—particularly Janet Crane and MaryAnne Holowaty. Over the years, they have encouraged me and survived my trials and errors.

I'm grateful, too, to Regina Ryan and Paul Deutschman, who knew there was a book in the tools concept and got me thinking about it; Marcelle Clements, who helped me organize my thoughts; Rick Isaacson, who took me by the hand and made this book happen; Mark Reiter, who made the way easy; the entire Rodale crew, who graciously put up with my last-minute changes; and most of all, Julia VanTine, my editor at Rodale, who made this book come alive.

I also want to thank my friends, who listened to me drone about this book for many months, and my aunts and uncle, who I know will add this book to their shelf of works written by famous relatives.

There has been no stronger influence in my life than my father, Elliott Nonas, who has taught me much about writing and who will always be my favorite poet. Thank you, Dad. Thanks also to my brother, Adam, who always believed in me, and to my children. They gave me space to write and lovingly never doubted that this book would get finished.

And, finally, many, many thanks to the patients at the VanItallie Center. They have taught me about vigilance and what it means to try and try again, with humor, passion, and unending optimism. Because of them, I know people can succeed at managing their weight. Because of them, this book exists.

—C.N.

Part 1

GETTING STARTED

The French Paradox, American-Style

Maybe you've heard of the French Paradox. Despite eating tons of saturated fat and smoking like chimneys, the French have traditionally had an extraordinarily low rate of heart disease.

Here in the States, we have our own health puzzle. Call it the American Paradox.

At any one time, up to 40 percent of women and up to 24 percent of men are on a diet. But almost 51 percent of women—and almost 60 percent of men—are overweight, while 22 percent of American men and women are obese!

That's not all. Some experts predict that if our level of obesity continues to climb at the current rate, theoretically *every man and woman in this nation will be overweight* by the year 2030.

How can this be? There are no simple answers. Overweight and obesity are complex conditions with many causes. But in my view, the American Paradox isn't such a puzzle after all. We eat too much, move too little, and look for easy solutions.

The question is: How did we get this way?

Modern Life: A Nonstop Buffet

Our culture may exalt bikini-ready bodies, but our lifestyle promotes obesity. Consider what we're up against.

Modern conveniences. Where would we be without our SUVs, washing machines, remote controls? We'd be a lot lighter, most likely. Because the easier life gets, the fatter *we* get. No one breaks a sweat pressing buttons or flicking switches.

Here's just one example of how machine power has replaced muscle power. A hundred years ago, muscle power by actual people supplied

30 percent of the energy used in farm and factory work. Today? One percent.

TV. If you're the typical American, your TV is on a staggering 7 hours, 40 minutes per day. Research has shown that folks who watch 3 or more hours of TV a day are more than twice as likely to be fat as those who watch less than 1 hour. No surprise there. Flicking the remote burns about the same amount of calories as sleeping and eats up time we might spend in more active pursuits. But at least we don't snack when we snooze.

The "super-size it!" mentality. America: Home of the Free and Land of the Value Meal. The portions restaurants serve are staggering. When nutritionists from the Center for Science in the Public Interest in Washington, D.C., compared restaurant portions of 18 foods with the government's official serving sizes, they found:

■ A typical restaurant tuna salad sandwich weighs more than 10 ounces and packs 720 calories. The government's tuna sandwich? Four ounces and 340 calories.

■ A McDonald's super-size fries is 6 ounces and contains 540 calories. An official serving: 3 ounces and 220 calories.

■ A standard 3-cup serving of unbuttered popcorn has 160 calories. A small tub of movie-theater popcorn packs 7 cups and 400 calories; a medium tub, 16 cups and 900 calories.

We can't lay all the blame at the feet of the restaurant industry, though. We serve up hefty portions at home, too.

The Diet Trap: From (Cabbage) Soup to Nuts

The "experts" who write those blockbuster weight-loss books tell us diets don't work (except for theirs, of course). They typically offer some incomprehensible scientific explanation for eating this and not that, along with lists of "good" foods to eat a lot of and "bad" foods to shun.

Technically, these experts are wrong. Diets *do* work—if you follow them. If you cut calories, you'll lose weight, whether you're eating pork rinds or baked potatoes.

WIGGLE MORE, WEIGH LESS?

You probably know people who eat whatever they want and don't gain an ounce. It may be because they never sit still. Literally.

Researchers at the Mayo Clinic in Rochester, Minnesota, measured the calorie burn of 17 women and 7 men doing six different things: lying down, sitting still, standing still, walking on a treadmill, fidgeting while seated, and fidgeting while standing.

What they found: The study participants burned ½ calorie more per minute when they fidgeted in their chairs than when they sat still. And they burned 1 full calorie more per minute when they fidgeted when standing up, compared with standing still.

The researchers hypothesized that "nonexercise activity thermogenesis," or NEAT—a fancy term for fidgeting—caused the increased calorie burn.

Half a calorie a minute may not seem like much. But consider this: If you sit at a desk for 8 hours a day, you could burn up to 300 calories more by tapping your hand or foot or swinging your arms or legs, as these folks did. And if you can burn an extra 300 calories a day, you could lose about 30 pounds a year!

My advice: Play as much footsie as you can.

Here's the rub. Shedding a few pounds quickly on a fad diet is easy. But continuing to lose and then maintaining that loss? That's hard.

And that's what these experts don't tell you. We can't eat cabbage soup or 10-ounce steaks every day for the rest of our lives. Or deny ourselves the foods we love. Or eat our meager meals in the basement so our families can eat their meat loaf and mashed potatoes in peace.

So why do we continue to buy into every fad diet that comes down the pike? Because somewhere along the way, we've confused the word "dieting" with "diet."

The word "diet" comes from the Greek *diaita*, or "manner of living." In the most literal sense, a diet is a way of life.

But that's not the way most of us understand the word.

To most of us, diets are a temporary affair in which we suffer for a set amount of time—a week, a month, a year. The longer we suffer, the more weight we lose.

But after a while, we can't suffer anymore. At that point, the question is: Now what? How else do we lose pounds or maintain our weight, if not by depriving ourselves? After all, we can't eat like people of normal weight.

And so, because we're no longer "dieting," we return to our old ways. The sad truth is, while we know how to gain and lose weight, we don't know how to lose it once and for all.

There's no doubt in my mind that we'd be more successful in our weight-loss efforts if we'd stop "dieting" and be faithful to the true meaning of "diet" by making our eating habits part of our everyday lifestyles.

Weight Loss for Keeps: Hope for Human Yo-Yos

I try to offer my clients healthy lifestyle adjustments they can live with. In this book, I offer the same to you. Your lifestyle encompasses your eating habits, level of activity, and behavior as well as the way you think about and talk to yourself.

Just as important, I'd like to help prevent you from returning to your old lifestyle—the one that made and kept you fat.

I won't lie: This is easier said than done. Evidence from clinical weight-loss studies suggests that few people who lose weight are able to keep it off.

And yet, there's hope. More recent research has found that more people than originally thought do successfully maintain their weight loss—and have done so for years.

The National Weight Control Registry (NWCR) is the largest study to date of what are called weight-loss maintainers. The typical NWCR participant has lost an average of 66 pounds and has kept a minimum of 30 pounds off for 5 years. Just under half lost the weight on their own. The researchers involved in this study conduct painstaking

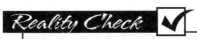

THE SNACKWELL'S SYNDROME

Remember when low-fat baked goods hit the store shelves? I do. Because that was around the time we started believing we could eat as much low-fat anything as we wanted.

When, despite our low-fat mania, our waistlines continued to expand, we started to get the message that low-fat cookies, muffins, chips, and cheese weren't a weight-watcher's best friends. Fact is, reducing fat helps you lose weight only if you cut calories, too. And unfortunately, low-fat foods can pack the same number of calories—or even more calories—as the fat-laden real thing. (Manufacturers of low-fat foods often compensate for the loss of flavor and texture that comes from a lower fat content by adding sugar.)

Consider:

- One regular fig bar packs 50 calories. So does one fat-free fig bar.

- Three regular chocolate chip cookies contain 160 calories. Three of the reduced-fat kind contain 150 calories.

- One cup of regular chicken noodle soup has 120 calories. A cup of the reduced-fat version has 140 calories.

The bottom line? Calories do count. So count them up.

---

analyses of their maintainers' eating habits, behavior, and lifestyle to figure out how—and why—they succeed where others don't.

But NWCR participants aren't the only weight-loss maintenance success stories. In another study of 500 people in the general population, among those who intentionally lost 10 percent or more of their weight, 47 to 49 percent kept it off for at least 1 year, and 25 to 27 percent shed it for 5 or more years.

We know that, for the most part, all of these people eat low-fat diets, get a significant amount of exercise, and keep food diaries. (More about that in a later chapter.)

The question is: How do weight-loss maintainers get themselves to do what they need to do, day after day, month after month, year after year? Researchers are still studying that very question. But it's very likely that these people have discovered the incredible power of tools.

Putting Tools to Work for You

Lifestyle change is *the* determinant of whether or not people will lose weight and maintain that loss, according to Yale University's Kelly Brownell, Ph.D., a foremost expert in eating and weight disorders. Dr. Brownell defines "lifestyle change" as altering our eating and exercise behaviors as well as our attitudes and emotions.

There's no denying it: Change is hard, even painful. But there's something that can make it easier.

Tools.

In working with thousands of overweight men and women throughout the years, I'm convinced that one of the main secrets to successful weight loss and weight-loss management (what I've dubbed weight control) is to learn to use what I call tools—practical, common-sense strategies that help keep your eating and exercise habits on track in virtually any situation.

When a computer repairperson or car mechanic dips into his stash of tools, he knows exactly which ones will get the job done and which will work in a pinch.

The tools in this book will help you master *your* job: to lose weight or maintain your weight loss. When you reach into your own personal cache of tools—tools *you* choose, based on your unique temperament and lifestyle—you know you'll find the ones to withstand a craving, to say no to an extra-large popcorn at the movies, or to stay in control at the buffet table. And if one tool doesn't always work, you have hundreds more to try. In fact, this whole book is a tool!

When you attempt to change problematic behaviors—in this case, overeating and physical inactivity—it's often best to take baby steps. Tools fit the bill; they're small and simple. And yet, using even one can help get and keep you at your goal weight for life. What's more, if you gain a few pounds or otherwise get into trouble, your tools can repair the problems.

10 Ways to Keep Lost Weight Lost

10. Periodically measure your portions to make sure they are what you think they are.

9. Throw away the remote and other energy-saving devices around your home and office.

8. Eat in only one room of the house. It should be a room with a table—and no television.

7. Eat slowly.

6. Increase your veggie intake. Fill half your dinner plate with vegetables, the other half with meat and starch (rice, potatoes, etc.).

5. Move more often and regularly.

4. Think of "diet" as a healthful revamping of your lifestyle, not a temporary period of deprivation.

3. Don't serve others food you wouldn't eat yourself. (It will be healthier for you and remove the temptation to enjoy the undesirable food with them!)

2. Strategize for a year: for every season, holiday, vacation, weekend, weekday. Put your strategies on wallet-size cards, laminate the cards, and carry them with you.

1. Reevaluate your tools regularly. Do they still support your goals? Can you add others to your tool kit?

You'll learn more about tools later in this book. For now, you need know only one thing: The hundreds of tools in this book have helped my clients not only to reach their goal weights but also to maintain them. I'm convinced that they can help you, too.

Of course, tools aren't magic. For any tool to be effective, it has to be usable.

Only you can decide whether a tool will help you attain or maintain

REDEFINING "SNACK"

Many people view a snack as an indulgence that falls outside the boundaries of good nutrition. But might you challenge this view? Consider this alternative definition of "snack."

- It's smaller than a meal.

- It should consist of the same kinds of nutritious foods you eat at mealtime, but it's eaten between meals. It should help complete the nutritional picture of your day.

- It's a planned part of your daily food plan.

- It's eaten to appease physical hunger. Period.

Write down *your* definition of a snack.

_____

_____

Now, answer the following questions.

Is your definition different from the one above? If so, what are the differences?

_____

_____

Do your snacks match any of the criteria above? If not, list the ways that your snacks differ.

_____

_____

Finally, could you use any of the criteria above to modify your snacking habits? For example, could you make all of your snacks smaller than a meal? Plan your snacks instead of eating them spontaneously? Snack on only low-calorie, healthy food?

_____

_____

a healthy weight—and how many tools you can comfortably wield at a time. It's better to commit to changing just one behavior (say, giving up bread and butter at dinner) than to attempt many changes that, deep down, you know you can't stick with for the long haul.

Identifying those tools that work for you—and picking the right ones for the job—takes practice. Fortunately, I'll streamline the selection process so you can start using them right away. You'll soon have enough tools to help you master your personal "Diet Danger Zones"—the specific situations that typically keep you from achieving diet and exercise success or lead to lapses, causing you to fall off the weight-control wagon.

That's why tools can succeed where diets fail. I'm not going to tell you what you can and can't eat. That's your affair. I'll give you diet-success *strategies*—hundreds of them—to get self-defeating eating and exercise behaviors back on track. You can use them in tandem with any diet plan, in virtually every situation, no matter what your age, habits, or lifestyle.

Let's Get Started!

There are two ways you can use this book. Choose the option that most appeals to you.

Option 1: Follow my simple, three-step process.

1. **Get ready . . .** Take the Eating Assessment Test (EAT) on page 35 to help you figure out where you are in your current eating and exercise habits.

2. **Get set . . .** From your EAT, determine your primary Diet Danger Zone: the People Zone, the Places Zone, or the Feelings Zone. (You may find that you fit into more than one zone, depending on the situation.)

3. **Go!** You're now ready to attack your personal Diet Danger Zones. Turn to part 3 (page 157) to find and learn about your unique Diet Danger Zone(s). At the top of the page, look for the numbered tool(s)

"SETTING FOOD POLICIES HELPED ME OUTWIT MY WEIGHT"

In 1998, Ronnie Silverman, at 5 feet 5 inches, weighed 210 pounds.

Then she discovered tools.

She now weighs in at 139 pounds and has kept off 70 of those original 80 pounds for 3 years.

"For me, tools provide a structure—something you can draw upon in challenging situations," says the 32-year-old urban planner.

For Silverman, those challenges include stress and social occasions, such as parties and vacations, in which she can't get healthy, low-calorie food—or, she concedes, she just doesn't want to.

Silverman's primary tool is to set "food policies"—rules about what she will and will not eat or do that are absolutely nonnegotiable.

While food policies sound rigid, they work for Silverman.

"If you have a food policy in those Diet Danger Zone situations, it prevents the danger from happening," she says. "If I set the policy before I enter the situation, I've made a decision, and there's no wavering."

For example, Silverman used to raid the bread basket in restaurants. She subsequently developed a food policy of taking no more than one piece. "It was not an option to take another," she says. Another food policy: She never

"prescribed" for that Diet Danger Zone. Then turn to part 2 (page 81) to look up the number of each particular tool.

Voilà! You now have a customized prescription to help you master your unique Diet Danger Zones.

Option 2: Use the freestyle approach.

If you're more of a browser or if you want support in starting or con-

brings "dangerous" foods into her house. So if she wants chips or cereal—her favorite treats—her policy is to buy a single-serving package and enjoy it.

Silverman, an avid runner, has also set an exercise policy: No more than 3 days can pass without her getting in a run or other form of exercise unless she's ill or has extenuating circumstances.

"This was a critical policy for me, especially when I was in the weight-loss phase," says Silverman. "I started running a couple of months into my program, and in 2000, I ran my first marathon."

Silverman's main piece of advice: "Don't pick a tool that *sounds* like a great idea but that doesn't fit with your lifestyle." So if you love cheese, don't give it up, even if you think you "should" because it's high in fat.

Instead, institute a "cheese policy," says Silverman. You might eat cheese only when you dine out or enjoy it in moderation once a week.

"Telling yourself that you're never going to have an Oreo cookie again doesn't make sense," says Silverman. "I had to figure out what my biggest diet 'potholes' were and then pick tools that addressed them but that were also simple for me to do. For tools to work, they have to mesh with your needs and your personality or your food issues."

tinuing a healthier lifestyle, simply page through the tools section and select the ones that appeal to you or seem to best fit your needs.

The browsing approach also works well if you're completely paralyzed in your weight-control efforts. When you feel completely derailed, browsing these tools may help jump-start your motivation. And if you can choose just one tool to try—no matter how small—you've taken a step toward regaining control.

Exchange Your FATitudes
for FITitudes

Sometimes, we focus so much on what we put into our mouths that we give no thought to the stuff in our heads that can sabotage our attempts to lose weight. Truth is, losing weight and keeping it lost require making dramatic changes in the way we think and—most important—in how we *act*.

In this chapter, we'll examine the common but often hidden thoughts, attitudes, and feelings that have kept many of us from losing weight or maintaining our weight loss in the past. I call them FATitudes.

If you can't seem to stay on track with a diet and exercise program, even when you very much want to lose weight, there's a good chance that FATitudes are derailing your efforts. FATitudes can be as basic as "I'm not losing weight quickly enough" or as complex as "I don't deserve to succeed." How FATitudes develop is beyond the scope of this book. But they typically take root when we're quite young and are the result of a complex psychological process we're often not aware of.

Fortunately, it's possible to exchange FATitudes for FITitudes: thoughts, beliefs, and behaviors that support the twin goals of healthful eating and regular exercise. You might consider FITitudes your "guiding lights"—truths that will help center you when you've gotten offtrack.

Once you start thinking about food and weight loss differently, your behavior will change, too—for the better.

I once had a client who loved baked potatoes. When they were available, she'd eat them until she was ready to burst.

Finally, she learned to eat just one. I asked her how. Her reply: "One was never enough, but neither were two or three. So I finally figured out that I might as well have just one."

Now, *that's* a FITitude.

The 10 Commandments
of Maintaining a Healthy Weight

10. Thou shalt define "success" as a modest weight loss tied to a healthy lifestyle.

9. Thou shalt occasionally allow yourself to have so-called forbidden foods. (Labeling any food "good" or "bad" is a major FATitude.)

8. Thou shalt keep the food diary or journal of your choice.

7. Thou shalt confront relapses or weight gain *immediately*. First, by admitting that you've lapsed. Second, by doing something about it, by grabbing a tool.

6. Thou shalt not use the words "should," "must," or "can't" in connection with food or weight.

5. Thou shalt lose weight or maintain your weight loss for *you*, not for anyone else.

4. Thou shalt preplan for events and emotions associated with overeating—social gatherings, stress, anger—and devise specific strategies for dealing with these situations.

3. Thou shalt learn when to eat rigidly (say, when you're confronting a Danger Zone, in which letting go may lead to major overeating) and when to loosen up (for example, if you usually don't eat egg yolks, but you're in a restaurant that doesn't offer Egg Beaters, your life won't fall apart if you decide to eat a whole egg).

2. Thou shalt use nonfood rewards to soothe or comfort yourself.

1. Thou shalt record specific portions in your food diary, rather than estimate them.

To Downsize Your Hips, Start with Your Head

FATitudes are like viruses. We can't see them, but they infect us all the same. And we suffer from their invisible assault.

It's absolutely crucial to put our FATitudes under the microscope, so to speak. If they remain hidden, they wield awesome power. But if we can see them, we can fight them—and come that much closer to managing them.

To help you identify your FATitudes, I've compiled a list of some of the most common ones, along with their polar-opposite FITitudes. (My list is by no means comprehensive. While your FATitudes may be completely different, they're just as destructive.)

FATitude: You think you can—and should—be "perfect." Consider the following statements.

"I was good all day . . . then I ate those Oreos. I've blown it now!"

---

this just in...

MAINTAINING GETS EASIER WITH TIME

The longer you're able to maintain your weight loss, the easier and more pleasurable it gets.

That's according to a study conducted by Drs. James Hill and Rena Wing, the founders of the National Weight Control Registry (NWCR). The NWCR is a group of more than 2,000 people who have lost at least 30 pounds and kept it off for at least a year. These doctors study them to find out how they've managed to do it.

Along with their colleagues, Drs. Hill and Wing asked 758 women and 173 men enrolled in the NWCR to fill out questionnaires that asked them to assess their feelings about their weight-loss maintenance routines. All of the people surveyed had kept off their weight for 2 years or more.

Those who'd kept their weight off longest said they had an easier time maintaining their new, lower weight than did those who'd maintained their loss for shorter periods. Moreover, they gave a higher rating to the pleasure they derived from staying slim than to the amount of effort it took.

"I should have lost more than a pound this week. I totally screwed up!"

"I didn't do my 45-minute walk today. This is the beginning of the end."

Any of this sound like you? If so, you may be caught in the sticky web of perfectionism—the belief that if you don't "do" dieting flawlessly, you might as well not do it at all.

Perfectionists feel that no matter how hard they try, their best is never good enough. And while perfectionism may make you a star boss or employee, it's bound to make you a washout when it comes to weight loss. That's because in weight loss, as in life, there's no such thing as "perfect." Eating a few too many cookies after dinner is nothing to jump off a building about—or to sabotage your weight-loss efforts over either.

One of my clients, Howard, finally shed the perfectionist FATitude. While he has regained 10 of his 60 lost pounds, he's kept off those remaining 50 pounds for 3 years. How? He finally learned that "slips" happen. When they do, he doesn't let them rattle him. He faces them head-on, acknowledges that he's not perfect, and gets back on track as fast as he can.

FITitude: You turn lapses into learning experiences. Ever heard of Jamie Clark, the young Canadian mountain climber who didn't make it to the top of Mount Everest? Twice?

The first time, Clark and his team "failed" 3,000 feet from the top.

The second time—2½ years later—they "failed" by the length of two city blocks.

The third time, Clark made it. And he credits his past "failures" for his ultimate triumph.

I love this story. It illustrates so perfectly the idea that success often comes once we learn the lessons contained in past failures. This same concept applies to weight-loss efforts.

There will be days you'll work your weight-control program perfectly. (Well, almost.) There will also be days when you return to your old ways. But if you can use past slipups to pinpoint what went wrong and devise ways to prevent them from recurring, chances are good that you'll ultimately succeed.

In fact, behind every weight-loss success story is what I call lapse experience. When you mean to eat a few potato chips from a bag but you eat a whole bag, eventually you learn that it's wiser to take one portion out of the bag, put the bag away, and then eat the one portion. (Or better yet, buy a one-serving bag.) Similarly, when you put off the gym for a few weeks but then go back, you have an opportunity to analyze why you stopped going and how you can keep from going AWOL again.

Don't deny or punish yourself for your lapses. Face them. Analyze them. Remember them. Learn from them. Eventually, they'll lead you to triumph.

FATitude: You equate "diet" with "deprivation." On most diets, foods become either "good" or "bad." And so do we, depending on how well we've stuck to an often extreme and unhealthy pattern of eating. This all-or-nothing attitude is a FATitude that sets you up to fail—especially if, crazed by deprivation, you say the heck with it and eat an entire pepperoni pizza.

FITitude: You equate "diet" with "health." When you adopt this FITitude, you realize that it's possible to enjoy food, rather than to fear it. A jelly doughnut ceases to be the root of all evil and becomes, once again, just a jelly doughnut. You come to view healthful eating not as a diet but as a way of life that affords you more energy, more vitality, and a better quality of life.

And yet you know that life without french fries would be bleak indeed. So you occasionally treat yourself to your favorite so-called forbidden foods when you feel these foods are worth it.

FATitude: You believe weight loss is an emotional cure-all. Some people believe that they'll lead charmed lives the minute they hit their goal weights. Think about it: Do *you* believe that you'll meet the right person, land a better job, or be happier, more creative, more popular, whatever, when the needle on the scale reaches a certain number?

A woman I once worked with said she was sure she'd meet "The One" once those extra pounds were gone. As gently as I could, I explained that while she could expect better physical health and improved

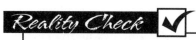

"DIET BARS" OR FAT TRAPS?

Do you reach for a chewy, chocolaty, granola-y "diet bar" to replace a meal?

Better take a second look at the label.

Nutritionally speaking, many diet bars are not much better for you than a candy bar, according to the Center for Science in the Public Interest (CSPI), a consumer group based in Washington, D.C.

CSPI recently analyzed the nutritional value of 86 kinds of cereal, snack, and diet bars. Just five earned its "Best Bite" award. (To win, a bar could contain only whole grains, provide at least 2 grams of fiber, and contain no more than 1 gram of saturated fat and 14 grams of sugar.)

Some of the diet bars that were evaluated—many of which sport the name of a specific diet plan—contained double the calories, twice the sugar, and nearly as much fat as another snack bar marketed as being diet-friendly!

Many are also laden with fat. One brand contains from 10 to 13 grams of fat, 3 to 8 of them artery-clogging saturated fat! Another contains from 6 to 7 grams of fat, 2 to 4 of them saturated fat.

Might I make a suggestion? Consider replacing these meal-replacement bars with a real meal. Or at least make sure you're using them as meal replacements. If you're eating them on top of meals, you might as well have a Snickers bar.

quality of life, there was no guarantee that, in losing weight, she'd find the perfect partner. (There's that word "perfect" again.) She got angry and left. I never saw her again.

Conversely, you may believe that reaching your goal weight will change your life so drastically that you panic and sabotage your weight-control program—the opposite side of the same coin. Yes, change involves risk. But are you willing to forgo that risk to the detriment of your physical health and personal growth?

FITitude: You value and nurture yourself, regardless of your weight. Your life doesn't begin when you reach your goal weight. After all, what happens if you want to lose 50 pounds but lose only 20? Does that mean you should put off going to Paris, signing up for that fiction-writing or pottery-throwing class, or searching for a more challenging job until you lose 30 more pounds?

Come on. Life is precious. Live it to the fullest, regardless of what the scale says.

FATitude: You're in a rush to lose the weight. Insisting that you *have* to lose 5 pounds a week—that it's not good enough to lose 2 (or not gain)—is a major FATitude. When you hold this attitude, you're focusing on the end result and missing out on the process. And it's going through the process—learning what works and doesn't work for you, trying new tactics, learning patience—that tends to make weight loss stick.

I once had a client who had lost a lot of weight, only to regain most of it. She finally came back to see me. She followed the diet I gave her for a week and lost 2 pounds.

Two pounds?! She was livid. She didn't see that she hadn't been able to follow any diet before this point and that even losing *no* weight would have been a triumph because she had stopped *gaining*. She left my office and never came back. This "I must lose it yesterday" FATitude is a perfect way to gain another 30 pounds!

Let's say you have 60 pounds to lose, and after a year, you've lost 15. You'd probably be frustrated and angry that you hadn't shed every last pound. But when was the last time you could say you lost 15 pounds for more than a few months? And even if it takes you another year to lose another 15 pounds, the fact remains: You'll have lost a significant amount of weight and kept it off. That's an incredible achievement.

FITitude: You're in it for the long haul. Understanding that weight loss takes time and that weight maintenance is a lifetime commitment is one of the most important FITitudes there is. People with this attitude aren't distraught if they don't lose weight every week or if they don't lose a lot of weight in a given week, even if they've worked their program diligently. After all, what's the hurry? They have come to view weight loss or weight maintenance as a lifestyle change, rather than as a temporary state of affairs. They have the rest of their lives to shed those extra pounds.

FATitude: You believe your eating is out of control. Many a client has wailed this to me. But it's pure FATitude. The reality was that their eating was typically out of control during a certain *time period*—maybe in the midafternoon or at night or during weekends. Rarely was their eating out of control from the time their alarm clocks went off.

I'll tell you what I tell them. Beating yourself up for being out of con-

THE INNER THINNESS INVENTORY

HOW MUCH IS JUST RIGHT?

There's a brand of potato chip whose catchphrase used to be "bet you can't eat just one." Many of us have a just-can't-say-when food, too. One bite somehow becomes the whole box, bag, or container.

If you struggle with controlling how much you eat of a certain food, using the "Just Right" tool may help. This tool has helped many of my clients satisfy their desires for their favorite foods yet remain in control of their eating.

Here's a sample "Just Right" table. After you've checked out the example, fill in the rest of the chart with the foods that tempt you.

Food	How Much Is Too Much?	How Much Is Too Little?	What Are My Options?
Häagen-Dazs ice cream	½ gallon	1 scoop	One double-scoop ice cream cone; 4 low-calorie fudge pops

trol is useless—and gives you a wonderful reason to eat yourself into oblivion. To battle this FATitude, analyze when these out-of-control periods usually occur (ideally, with the help of a food diary), find tools that help you cope during this time, and focus your efforts on just that time period.

FITitude: You keep a food diary. Self-monitoring—the systematic observation and recording of behaviors—has been called the most effective technique in the behavioral treatment of weight problems. Study after study has shown that keeping track of how much you eat and exercise is the key to losing weight and keeping it off.

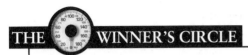

THE WINNER'S CIRCLE

"TOOLS AREN'T ONE SIZE— THEY'RE CUSTOM MADE FOR *YOU*"

A client of Cathy's since 1994, Donna Herman has lost 135 pounds. But "it's been an up-and-down ride," she says, ending with her gastric surgery in 1999.

But while she opted for surgery, the New York City resident, who works for a large corporation in Manhattan, says that learning to use tools has dramatically changed her perspective on weight loss.

"One problem with just about every other weight-loss method is that it's *one tool*," says Herman, 47. "But no one diet, no one plan will work for you for the rest of your life. What works for you today may not work for you tomorrow."

That's the beauty of tools, she says. They're not one size fits all but custom made for *you*. And there are a lot of them to choose from.

"Tools give you a whole arsenal of ways to avoid overeating in a specific situation," says Herman. "This arsenal is at your beck and call, and you can change the arsenal as your needs change."

Before she began to use tools, Herman says she often felt so guilty about overeating that she'd abandon her program. But now that she can *anticipate* the events that may trigger her urge to overeat and has tools to fight them, she's seldom caught unawares. "Tools allow you to plan a course of action that can help you avoid, modify, or lessen the ill effects of that urge," says Herman.

For example, a group that kept detailed food diaries during a 15-week study lost 64 percent more weight than those who didn't. Another study found that, out of 10 ways to change eating habits, self-monitoring was the only one that allowed people to keep off lost weight for 1½ years.

Keeping a running daily tab of everything you put into your mouth lets you literally see what you're doing right and what needs improvement. The insights you get from keeping a running account of your food intake will help keep you from gaining, or gaining back, unwanted pounds.

Herman calls herself a volume eater, "which simply means that I want a lot of food. For me, it's all about being filled up." She found that visualizing her hunger using a scale that rates fullness was quite helpful, using it to rate both her degree of hunger and her degree of satisfaction after eating.

"It was a revelation to discover when I was actually hungry or to determine when I'd had enough to eat—when I was satisfied instead of stuffed," she says.

While Herman regularly tries and discards tools, she does use one religiously.

"The one tool that always, always works for me—and I can't always get myself to use it because I know it works—is keeping food records," she says. "Writing down what I eat forces me to be conscious of when and what I'm eating. And that awareness generally results in my losing weight."

If you're new to the tool game, Herman has some pointers. "One, don't be afraid to discard a tool," she says. "When it doesn't work anymore, toss it and move on.

"Two, it's valuable to explore a tool that you have an immediate aversion to—the one that you just don't want or 'can't' try. It's interesting to figure out why you have the aversion to it—and why you may want to try it after all."

Moving Your Mind from Fat to Fit

There's no magical step-by-step process that will change your FATitudes to FITitudes. You'll need to consciously learn to think about food, your body, and weight loss in new ways. And those lessons aren't always learned instantly, in a flash of light.

But if you're willing to learn, the lessons will come.

I worked with a longtime client who kept gaining and losing weight over and over again. She was desperate.

I finally said to her, "Look, I'm not doing you any good. There's this 6-week program on body image, run by a legitimate therapy institute. Check it out, then come back."

Six weeks passed. When she returned, she said, "Cathy, I've had an epiphany!"

"Really!" I said, thrilled. "What is it?"

"I should eat only when I'm hungry!"

Now, I had told her that very same thing, probably dozens of times. But this time, she actually *heard* it. Who knows why. The point is, she didn't give up. She was willing to try a new approach. She was willing to try, period.

Most likely, changes in your thoughts, behaviors, and attitudes will occur gradually. But with each small success, each time you make a change that works, you become more aware of what works for you. Over time, these changes will become automatic.

One of the best ways to defeat the FATitudes that lurk within your head is to employ tools. In fact, knowing the tools that work for you—and using them—is a prime example of a FITitude. Whether you use tools every day or only in high-risk situations, they will help you overcome the negative thoughts and actions that otherwise could sabotage your weight-control efforts. And when you choose to use tools to defeat your FATitudes, you are making a statement that your health matters more than the offerings on any buffet table.

There are literally hundreds of tools available. You just have to keep trying them until you identify those that work best for you. Trust me: They are out there.

In the next chapter, I'll help you find them.

It's Tool Time!

■ Sam, a 45-year-old physician, finally broke his habit of eating nothing during the day and overeating at night. He has his assistant order him a healthy, low-calorie breakfast and lunch that he eats at his desk—and he's losing those extra pounds.

■ Susan, 40, an attorney, used to eat lunch at her desk, work late into the evening, and arrive home ravenous. Once she began to eat a healthy snack at noon and "lunch" at 4:00 P.M., her late-night eating fests stopped.

■ Mary, 35, who dines out as often as twice a day, now divides one of her typical restaurant meals in two. She eats an appetizer and salad at one meal and only the entrée at the other—and her dress size is dropping.

■ Sally, 29, knows she shouldn't nibble in front of the TV, but she's not willing to give it up. She is, however, willing to change the way she snacks. She noshes air-popped popcorn or another low-calorie snack from a huge bowl—using chopsticks to slow her down.

My clients all had eating behaviors that contributed to their weight problems. In each case, they changed one small behavior but reaped big benefits. These behavior-changing actions, called tools, have helped them shed from 10 to 100-plus pounds—and keep them off.

The Right Tools for the Job

As we saw in the first chapter, we live in a fat-promoting environment. Food is cheap and plentiful, and physical activity is at an all-time low. To achieve or maintain our goal weights, then, we must put buffers between us and that environment. Tools are these buffers.

A tool is an action that helps us monitor or change our weight-loss or weight-control behaviors. It can be as basic as measuring out portions or as ingenious as placing a piece of string across the entrance to the kitchen after dinner to discourage nighttime nibbling. Some tools are like those fire extinguishers encased in glass to be broken in case of emergency: They can save you when your eating threatens to rage out of control.

Tools can help us eat less, move more, and come to view ourselves, our weight, and food in healthier ways.

One thing tools aren't, however, is one size fits all. No matter how well a tool works for your friend or colleague, if you don't want to go there, it's not the tool for you.

Take food records, for example. There's no doubt that they make us more aware of our eating habits and that people who keep them tend to lose more weight and keep it off. But the traditional way to keep a food record—measuring portions, recording food as you eat it, looking up calorie amounts—may be too much work for you. Simply jotting down the number of times you eat during the day might suffice for you.

A successful tool—that is, a tool that works *for you*—is two things.

It's doable. For every tool that won't work for you, there's one that will. While keeping a traditional food journal may turn you off, you may find that a simpler type of record—and there are dozens of different types—keeps you on track. (More on food diaries in a minute.)

It's effective. Say you start keeping that food journal, but after a reasonable period of time, you're still eating 3,000 calories a day. Obviously, for you, this tool doesn't act as a deterrent to overeating. So you'll need to search for another tool or tools that will.

The Four Tool Groups

Remember learning about the Four Food Groups back in elementary school? The concept was that if you ate the appropriate amounts of food from all four groups (meat, dairy, grains, and fruits and veggies), you'd be eating a balanced diet. (The Basic Four morphed into the Food Guide Pyramid in 1992.)

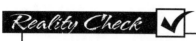

CARBS *DON'T* MAKE YOU FAT!

In recent years, books advocating low-carbohydrate, high-protein diets have been flying off bookstore shelves. They recommend consuming a diet that derives most of its calories from protein, such as meat and cheese, and significantly fewer calories—or none at all—from carbohydrates, such as bread, pasta, fruits, and most vegetables.

It's not surprising that, at first, many people are thrilled to follow a low-carb diet. After all, they get to eat double cheeseburgers, pork rinds, and creamy full-fat cheese. And their weight drops like a stone.

But that's not the whole story.

Low-carb diets can be extremely unhealthy. First, a low-carb diet is often high in fat. And high-fat diets can raise blood-cholesterol levels, thereby increasing the risk for heart disease and certain cancers.

Adding insult to injury, much of the initial weight loss that people experience is water, not fat.

Low-carbohydrate diets overwork the kidneys and can lead to dehydration, headaches, and fatigue (not to mention bad breath). And as ketones build up in your blood, your body may produce high levels of uric acid, which is a risk factor for kidney stones and gout, a painful swelling of the joints. Finally, ketosis can be very dangerous for people with diabetes.

Following a reduced-calorie diet that includes proteins, fats, and, yes, high-fiber carbohydrates is the best—and safest—way to lose weight and keep it off.

What I'd like you to do, as a person who wants to lose weight and keep it off, is to plan your eating around the Four Tool Groups. If you use tools from all four groups, you'll have a balanced weight-loss program. That's because these tools will help you with all the major components of weight-loss and maintenance success: your food selections and portions, your level of physical activity, your emotional relationship with food, and the way you choose to act in the face of temptation.

Food Tools

These tools help you manage your intake of calories and nutrients such as fats, carbohydrates (including fiber), and protein. Many of these tools automatically help you follow a low-fat, high-fiber diet—my personal prescription for weight loss. But you'll also find tools that help you follow virtually any diet plan, from Atkins to The Zone.

You'll also find tools to help you avoid weight-loss pitfalls you may not even know are affecting you. I call one of these pitfalls "portion drift."

I once worked with a woman who'd lost 80 pounds and kept it off for about a year. She was religious about following her chosen diet plan and each day took her diet lunch to work—rice and beans packed in a plastic storage container.

So when she gained 10 pounds, she couldn't figure out why. She wasn't eating any differently. Even studying her food diary didn't help.

Puzzled, I said, "Do me a favor. Start measuring out your portions."

She said, "I don't need to. I know exactly how much I'm eating—I eat the same thing almost every day."

"Just do it," I said.

It turns out that, yes, she was eating the same stuff. But then the lightbulb went on: For some reason, she'd begun to pack her rice-and-beans lunch more tightly into the container. In fact, she was eating a whole extra portion, which added up to hundreds of extra calories a day! Once she started measuring her portions, the extra weight started to come off.

Mood Tools

While food tools focus primarily on our physical selves, mood tools are designed to shape up our mental and psychological states. For example, you'll find lots of tools for reshaping negative thoughts about yourself and your body into more positive ones. These tools are critical to weight loss and weight-loss management. When your thoughts are supporting your weight-loss efforts, it becomes not only easier but more pleasant to follow a diet and exercise program.

The Top 10 Reasons to Use Tools

10. They give structure to your eating behaviors, making you feel more in control of your food choices and less of a slave to your cravings.

9. They make it easier to make "thin" choices in a fat-promoting environment.

8. They can help you to take action to improve your physical health, especially if you have high cholesterol or a chronic condition such as high blood pressure, heart disease, or diabetes.

7. They help keep you honest.

6. When your weight-loss program is falling apart or you've fallen off the maintenance wagon, they can help you get back on track.

5. They work in virtually every situation.

4. You can tailor tools to your unique lifestyle, situation, and needs.

3. You can use as few—or as many—as you want.

2. They help you think about yourself and your body in new, more positive ways.

1. They help take the emotion out of emotional eating. They teach you new ways to cope without food when you're lonely, angry, or stressed.

Move Tools

We all have different levels of physical ability, depending on our current weight and health condition. No matter what your level, though, the move tools will help you become more active, whether in everyday life or in starting and sticking with a more formal exercise program.

Here's one move tool that I love: If you work out at home, attach your TV remote control to a small piece of your exercise equipment, such as a resistance band or a 2-pound dumbbell. If you have a treadmill or stair-climber in your TV room, attach it to that. Every time you pick up the remote, you'll be reminded to get off the couch and into your exercise gear.

Behavior Tools

While the goal of mood tools is to reshape your thoughts, the aim of behavior tools is to change your behaviors—specifically, self-defeating behaviors that, unbeknownst to you, are sabotaging your weight-loss or maintenance program. These behaviors include everything from eating in the car to "awfulizing" overeating situations.

this just in...

BEHAVIOR "TOOLS" TO MAKE A DIFFERENCE

Feeling a bit skeptical about the power of tools? Consider this. People who use behavior-modification techniques in their weight-loss or maintenance programs are more apt to keep the pounds off than those who don't, according to a scientific paper coauthored by obesity expert John P. Foreyt, Ph.D., director of the Behavioral Medicine Research Center at Baylor College of Medicine in Houston.

In behavior modification, you consciously change eating and other behaviors that contribute to overweight. (Sounds a lot like using tools, doesn't it?) The five main techniques of behavior modification are:

1. Self-monitoring. You observe and write down your behavior, typically in a notebook kept just for that purpose. For example, you might keep a daily food diary or activity log or record changes in your weight or body fat.

2. Stimulus control. You identify and change "cues" that trigger overeating or inactivity. This might include eating only at the kitchen table, keeping no snack foods in the house, and placing your gym bag at the front door at night to remind you to exercise the next day.

While changing your behavior is hard, behavior tools can make it easier. I remember when one of my clients, Jane, once showed up for her appointment in distress.

"I've been bad," she said. "I wasn't going to come today." (She'd wanted to lose the weight she'd gained in between our visits before her next appointment. This seems as pointless to me as cleaning your house so your housekeeper won't think you're a slob.)

"Good to see you," I said. "Why were you 'bad'?"

"I've been eating everything that isn't nailed down."

"What do you have for breakfast?" I asked.

"Cheerios, fat-free milk, and a banana."

"What happens after breakfast?"

"I almost never eat between breakfast and lunch," she said.

---

3. Cognitive restructuring. You raise your awareness of negative thoughts about yourself and your body, then work to change those thoughts. (Many obese people suffer from low self-esteem and body-image problems.) For example, you could keep a "thought record," a kind of food diary for your brain. In it, you record specific upsetting situations, how you felt, what you thought, the evidence that supports (and also refutes) those thoughts, and a different, more balanced way to think about the situation.

4. Stress management. You learn and use specific techniques for reducing the stress in your life. (The more stress you're under, the more likely you are to overeat.) Examples of these techniques include meditation, progressive muscle relaxation, and deep breathing.

5. Social support. You find and maintain a network of family, friends, or groups you can turn to. For instance, you might include family members in your treatment program, participate in church or community-related activities, or join Weight Watchers, Overeaters Anonymous, or another group.

"What do you have for lunch?"

"Usually, a turkey sandwich."

So far, Jane didn't sound "out of control" to me. But then she said, "After work is when I really let go. Once I get home, I don't stop eating until I go to bed."

Although Jane felt that she was "bad" all day, the truth was that she was being "good" for the majority of the day. I suggested that Jane use the compartmentalization tool, in which you focus on the main problem—in Jane's case, night eating. When Jane used this tool, she focused just on that problem, brainstormed ways to solve it, and felt much better about herself. Identifying the problem and working to solve it makes it much less overwhelming and gives you a much-needed feeling of control.

But there's one more tool that you need to be aware of.

Writing Down the Pounds

Consider the mirror. Without having access to this everyday tool, many of us would sail through the day unaware of the spinach on our front teeth, the coffee stain on our blouses, or the unmentionable in our noses.

A food diary—a written record of the type and amount of food you consume each day—acts much like a mirror. It reflects a true picture of our eating selves, clearly and objectively pointing out our problem eating patterns and behaviors.

While we may not like what we learn, a food diary is a valuable tool because—like a mirror—it gives us the opportunity to correct the flaws we see.

If you've never kept a food diary, I ask that you be willing to try it now. As you'll see in The Ultimate Weight-Loss Weapon: A Pen (page 203), keeping a food diary is one of the most important weight-loss and weight-maintenance tools available. It can help you:

■ Track your intake of calories and other nutrients, such as fat and carbohydrates

TRY OUT A TOOL!

Turn to part 2 (page 81) and leaf through the four tool groups. Pick five tools that appeal to you from any group or groups. Write them here.

_____

_____

_____

_____

_____

Now, pick one tool you're willing to try right now. Use it at least three times. (Try the other tools, too, if you like, but you're committed to trying only one.)

When and where did you use the tool? Did it work? Did it flop? How did you feel when you put it into action? Record your experience here.

_____

_____

_____

_____

_____

_____

_____

_____

_____

_____

_____

_____

_____

- Become more aware of portion sizes

- Get a snapshot of your current eating patterns and behavior around food—the good, the bad, and the downright ugly

- Pinpoint lapses—when, how, and even why they happened

- See the connections between your mood and your food intake

There are dozens of ways to keep a food diary. But generally speaking, diaries can be broken down into three categories.

- The traditional diary, in which you record the food you eat, the amount you eat, and its calorie count. If you're an organized type who likes crunching numbers, this may be the diary for you.

- The "breakdown" diary, in which you record your intake of specific nutrients. Folks who choose these diaries may be on diets in which they must tally grams of fat and carbohydrates, or they may wish to improve their health by monitoring their intake of nutrients such as sodium or cholesterol.

- The feelings diary, in which you focus on why you overeat. You record not only what and how much you ate but why you ate it and how you felt after eating it. Emotional eaters often find this type of diary extremely helpful.

Some folks equate keeping a food diary with taking out the trash—a bothersome but necessary task. Others grow to love keeping their diaries.

One client told me that writing in her diary gave her a sense of accomplishment, much like a good workout can. She said, "Each time I make an entry, I know I've done something good for myself."

In my view, the food diary is the mother of all tools, no matter which one you use or how you use it. So as you use the hundreds of tools in this book, take advantage of one of the most effective.

The Eating Assessment Test (EAT)

Maps are wonderful things. I travel thousands of miles a year, giving lectures and presentations, and my sense of direction is feeble, to say the least. Without my stash of well-worn state maps and my trusty highway atlas, it's conceivable that I would be driving the Brooklyn-Queens expressway or the Los Angeles freeway until the end of time, unable to find my exit.

The point is, if you want to get somewhere you've never been, you rely on a map to tell you where you are and the route you need to follow. You might consider the series of thought-provoking questionnaires and tests that you're about to take—called the Eating Assessment Test (EAT)—as your personal road map to weight control. The EAT can help you figure out where you are in your eating and exercise habits at this moment and help you discover where you need to be. And like a map, it can keep you headed in the right direction. Whether you're beginning a new weight-loss program or you want to get your eating and exercise program back on track, the EAT can point the way.

This test isn't a one-time deal, though. It's designed to be used time and again, so you can continually monitor your progress, reevaluate your current weight-control program, and troubleshoot new and continuing issues. In fact, I suggest that you take it quarterly.

When you're feeling discouraged, unmotivated, or out of control, taking the EAT can help you see the big picture and help you refocus your efforts. Make several copies and keep them in a folder next to your food diary. Every 3 months, take out a copy and chart your progress. Keep all the copies; you'll want to look back on them in the future.

Have fun!

EAT #1

Find Your Hidden "Fat Traps"

IF you've been battling your weight for any period of time, you're well-aware of your personal diet Waterloos. This list is long: nighttime eating, chronic snacking, the inability to close a bag of Doritos and walk away.

Still, you may not be conscious of every self-defeating eating pattern that may be contributing to your extra pounds. I call these unconscious eating patterns fat traps. To shed those extra pounds once and for all—or to keep lost pounds lost—it's crucial to uncover those hidden snares.

An eating pattern is simply the number of times we eat in a day. This portion of the EAT is designed to make you see it in flashing neon lights. Many of my clients have completed this section and been amazed at how much they're actually eating!

1a. Indicate how many meals and snacks you eat on one average weekday by placing check marks in the blanks provided. If you have more than one snack between meals (or more than one taste, bite, or nibble), use a check mark for each one.

Breakfast _____

Midmorning snack(s) _____

Lunch _____

Midafternoon snack(s) _____

Dinner _____

Evening snack(s) _____

Daily tastes, bites, and nibbles _____

Next, do the same tally for one average weekend day.

Breakfast _____

Midmorning snack(s) _____

Lunch _____

Midafternoon snack(s) _____

Dinner _____

Evening snack(s) _____

Daily tastes, bites, and nibbles _____

1b. Add up your check marks and compare your eating patterns for weekdays and weekends.

Number of weekday meals _____

Number of weekend meals _____

1c. Then, to find the part of the day in which you tend to eat the most, tally the number of times you eat (include daily tastes, bites, and nibbles).

Between breakfast and lunch _____

Between lunch and dinner _____

After dinner _____

EAT #2
Identify Your Eating Behaviors

WHILE eating patterns pertain to the number of times you eat in a day, eating behaviors are where, when, and how you eat. The ways you act around food stem from many sources—your childhood, lifestyle, and habits, to name a few. Maybe you were raised on hearty home cooking and can't give it up, even though you know that a lot of it ends up on your backside. Or perhaps as you advanced in your career, getting to the gym wasn't a priority. Or could it be that you just let it all go when you got married or had kids?

Regardless of how or why you acquired your eating behaviors, one thing's for sure: Supportive ones help keep you at your ideal weight, and unsupportive ones threaten to make your jeans snugger than they should be.

Fortunately, once you become aware of the eating behaviors that hurt you, you can take steps to unlearn them.

For each question, estimate the number of times per week that you engage in the following:

1. How many times a week do I eat:

	TIMES/WEEK	TIMES/WEEKEND
a. At-home meals at the dining-room table?	_____	_____
b. At a restaurant?	_____	_____
c. At my desk?	_____	_____
d. Take-out food?	_____	_____
e. In front of the TV?	_____	_____
f. While standing up?	_____	_____

Read the list below and check the appropriate response.

2. Do I tend to eat less or more when:

	LESS	MORE
a. I drink alcohol?	_____	_____
b. I'm at a restaurant?	_____	_____
c. I'm at home?	_____	_____
d. Someone is watching me?	_____	_____
e. I've already overeaten?	_____	_____

EAT #3

Identify Your Eating Profile

YOUR eating habits and behavior are as unique as your fingerprints. And yet, the thoughts, beliefs, and emotions that underlie them can be strikingly similar for everyone. They're so similar that I've classified them into seven eating "profiles." Identifying your personal Eating Profile can help you recognize and confront unconscious eating behaviors that may be holding you back in your weight-loss efforts.

Read the Eating Profiles below, then select the *one* that you feel best describes you.

The Baby

Main characteristic: Not taking responsibility for what and how much you eat.

Favorite quote: "Everyone else can eat it. I want it too! I want what I want when I want it!"

Frequently seen: Stomping feet and flailing fists.

Mini-profile: Sometimes consciously, sometimes not, Babies believe that they should be able to eat like "everyone else." Or they believe that they're serving others' needs rather than their own when they accept others' invitations or exhortations to eat. Their behavior can masquerade as politeness. For example, at a family gathering, a Baby may think, "My Aunt Lucy went to all this trouble to prepare my favorite— lasagna. How could I be so rude as to turn down seconds?" While Babies can reel off everything they *haven't* eaten, they "forget" what they *have* eaten.

The Ostrich

Main characteristic: Denial and magical thinking.

Favorite quote: "I didn't eat all *that*." Variations: "I didn't/don't eat that much" or "I'll start my diet tomorrow."

Frequently seen: Shrugging shoulders and looking surprised. Avoiding the scale, believing that if they don't *see* their weight, they won't *be* their weight.

Mini-profile: Ostriches hide what they eat from others—and from themselves. They figure that if no one sees them eat it, then they haven't, in fact, eaten it. And if they "forget" that they've eaten a package of cookies in the car, then those calories can't be absorbed. Ostriches' lack of short-term food memory makes it difficult for them to keep food diaries. What's more, they devise intricate rules about what does and does not "count" when it comes to food. The phrase "It doesn't count if . . ." is an Ostrich catchphrase, as in: "It doesn't count if I eat in the car . . . off someone else's plate . . . out of the container. . . ."

The Restrained Eater

Main characteristic: Extremes of dieting and overeating.
Favorite quote: "I'll just have one."
Frequently seen: Wearing a pious expression.
Mini-profile: Restrained Eaters eat like birds in public, making everyone wonder, "How in the world can she eat like that and still be so heavy?" The answer: They're always on diets—often, a fly-by-night one—and their constant deprivation leads them to episodes of extreme overeating. When Restrained Eaters go off their plans, they do it in a big way. After all, they're going to start their diets tomorrow.

Restrained Eaters also tend to overeat on "diet" foods such as fat-free cheese or rice cakes. It's possible to eat a whole block of fat-free cheese and an entire box of fat-free crackers, a smidgen at a time.

The Slow Gainer

Main characteristic: Avoidance and poor impulse control.
Favorite quote: "I'm gaining half a pound a week, sometimes a couple of pounds in a month! I don't know how it happens. I don't eat that much."
Frequently seen: Stepping on the scale with optimism, then stepping off in shock.
Mini-profile: Many Slow Gainers' destructive eating behaviors are subtle—so subtle that to detect them would require some heavy food-diary analysis. Unfortunately, Slow Gainers rarely keep food diaries. And even if they did, they would probably neglect to write down everything that they put into their mouths—which is unfortunate, because Slow Gainers are slaves to food availability and their own impulses. They may decide to have a salad with blue cheese dressing because they haven't had it in so long or choose the garlic mashed potatoes because they "never"

do. They may also bake brownies or another high-calorie treat for the rest of the family and taste while they bake. Slow Gainers often feel victimized because they truly believe that they're doing everything they can to keep their weight down and that they should be rewarded, not punished.

The Weekend Eater

Main characteristic: Extremes of vigilance and abandon.

Favorite quote: "I eat well and exercise all week. But the weekend is my time for me!"

Frequently seen: Ordering salads and fruit cups Monday through Thursday and the mozzarella appetizers or spicy chicken wings with blue cheese dressing on Friday—and maybe even Saturday and Sunday.

Mini-profile: Weekend Eaters restrict their eating during the week, but once Friday night rolls around, watch out! These folks usually reserve their weekends for socializing and partying, and they can't enjoy themselves if they must monitor their alcohol intake, crunch calories during their Saturday dinner out, or not sample what they make during their Sunday afternoon cooking fest. But like those of us who don't balance the checkbook, Weekend Eaters end up paying the price—in extra pounds. It's hard to bank all your calories to "spend" on the weekend, and it's even more difficult to make up during the week for letting loose on the weekends.

The Good Fairy/Bad Fairy

Main characteristic: Using food as both a reward and a punishment.

Favorite quote: "I've been so good. I never eat ice cream, so today I can have some."

Frequently seen: Dutifully ignoring the cheesecake on a friend's kitchen counter, then cruising the bakery section of the supermarket for a slice. Or two.

Mini-profile: To Good Fairies/Bad Fairies, food is a double-edged sword. They view it as both a reward for a job well-done and as a punishment when they feel ashamed and guilty about overeating and its consequences. There's an inherent catch-22 in being a Good Fairy/Bad Fairy.

If you've been "good," you deserve the treat. But once you have it, you have to be punished for eating it. Punishment may include starving the next day or even abandoning a weight-loss plan.

The Stress Eater

Main characteristic: Anxiety, stress, or fear.
Favorite quote: Stress Eaters rarely talk. They eat.
Frequently seen: Zoning out in front of the television with a family-size bag of chips.
Mini-profile: To one degree or another, all of us are stress eaters who use food as a tranquilizer. Who hasn't turned to comforting, creamy ice cream or soft, velvety cheesecake to quell the tension caused by long work hours, demanding partners and children, endless bills, and a lack of downtime? (And if our favorite comfort foods aren't available, Jell-O—in powder form—or a few heaping tablespoons of peanut butter work just as well.) But while some people can exorcise stress by going for a walk, soaking in a bubble bath, or crawling into bed to read a few pages of a novel, Stress Eaters tend to turn to food *first* in an effort to anesthetize scary feelings.

EAT #4

Confront Your Inner Saboteur

WHAT makes your weight-loss efforts fail time and again? Why do you get to your goal weight or lose some weight, only to immediately pile the pounds back on? Blame the Inner Saboteur. Just when you take one step forward, this silent enemy—born of negative or distorted thoughts, feelings, and behaviors that may hark back to childhood—drags you two steps back, making you abandon your efforts for no discernible reason. That's why it's crucial to drag your Inner Saboteur out of the shadows.

This portion of the EAT illustrates the four types of Inner Saboteur. After reading all four, you may feel that you have more than one. While that may be true, choose the *one* saboteur that you suspect most undermines your weight-control efforts.

Inner Saboteur #1: The Traditionalist

Irrational belief: When it comes to dieting and weight loss, it's better to stick with the known—even when the known no longer works—than to experiment with the unknown.

Mini-profile: Traditionalists find it stressful to even consider changing their food choices or meal patterns. They stubbornly stick with the same diet or beliefs about weight loss, even when they fail. Why? Because they work. At least, they worked once. Traditionalists can also be stubborn about giving up behaviors that don't support their weight-loss attempts. For example, they *have* to have their two glasses of wine with dinner, or they refuse to give up their morning bagel for lighter fare.

Example: Five years ago, a Traditionalist had success with a particular fad diet. Ever since, she turns to that diet, ascribing to it powers that border on the mystical. She thinks, "The last time I was on this diet, I lost 30 pounds. The time before that, I lost 40!" The thing is, this time around, the diet is making her gain, not lose. It may be because it's hard to eat nothing but meat (or fruit or rice or hard-boiled eggs or what have you). Or it could be that when she "follows" a diet, she makes lots of substitutions. She has 6 ounces of tuna instead of 3 or a bagel with nothing on it instead of two slices of whole wheat toast.

Inner Saboteur #2: The Perfectionist

Irrational belief: If you can't "do" weight loss perfectly, don't do it at all.

Mini-profile: Perfectionists have an all-or-nothing way of looking at most things, including weight loss. And for this group, any deviation from their diet is a failure. For example, if, in a moment of weakness, they have a tablespoon of peanut butter from the jar or five marshmallows, the day is shot. Never mind that they followed their diet until 5:30 P.M.

That peanut butter or those marshmallows give them license to overeat the rest of the night. After all, they've ruined their perfect score.

Example: At a restaurant, the Perfectionist orders a salad. (Of course, she's grilled the waiter, making him swear that it won't contain meat or cheese, the dressing will come on the side, and the greens will be varied and not merely iceberg lettuce.) The salad arrives. She loses her cool: She forgot to ask to hold the croutons! She tries to pick them out, but they're so big and crunchy, she succumbs to their greasy appeal. As punishment for this transgression, she goes home and eats a dozen Oreos.

Inner Saboteur #3: The Rebel

Irrational belief: Food is a gift that you give yourself.

Mini-profile: Some people have problems with authority figures. In this case, Rebels view food as the authority figure—and they resent being "told what to do" by a diet plan. That's why they tend to exclaim, "The heck with it!" and defiantly break a diet.

Example: The Rebel has had a killer day. This morning, the scale said she'd gained 2 pounds, even though she'd followed her eating plan to the letter. The boss groused at her all day. Her kids were whiny and demanding when she picked them up from soccer practice. She's angry and drained: Nobody ever takes care of *her*. Damn the torpedoes—she's going to take care of herself! Instead, she takes care of three-quarters of an Entenmann's red-raspberry pastry.

Inner Saboteur #4: The Victim

Irrational belief: If you dare to assert your wants and needs rather than those of others, you'll lose their love and approval.

Mini-profile: Victims are never at fault for their self-defeating food choices or eating behavior. The blame belongs to everyone else—the food-pushing relative, the friend who ordered nachos at the movie, the partner who brings home junk food. (Even if the partner thoughtfully hides the junk, Victims can always find it.) Victims would be much thinner, they think, if others didn't always sabotage them. Unfortunately, while the blame sticks to everyone around them, the extra pounds always stick to them.

Example: At a business lunch, a Victim orders what his client orders—a grilled Reuben with a side of fries and slaw and a hot-fudge sundae. After all, why make the client uncomfortable by getting what he really wanted: a salad and fresh fruit for dessert? And why did he eat those five slices of bread and butter? He didn't want to inconvenience his guest by asking the waiter to remove the bread basket.

<u>EAT</u> #5
Take Stock of Your Support System

DO you have:

- A food-pushing friend?

- A colleague who's demonstrated quiet support for your weight-loss efforts by removing the candy jar from her desk?

- A sister who says, "Should you really be eating that?" each time you unfold your napkin?

- A partner who does the dinner dishes so you aren't tempted to nibble on leftovers?

These folks are your support system (or, in some cases, your *nonsupport* system). In this portion of the EAT, you'll do an exercise that helps you identify the people in your life who help or hinder your struggle with weight.

1. In the middle of a blank piece of paper, draw a circle that represents you.

2. Draw other circles around "you" that represent the important people in your life: spouse, kids, siblings, parents, friends, colleagues. Place them nearer or farther away from you depending on how much time you spend with them rather than how emotionally close you are to them.

3. Assign each a plus sign (+), minus sign (−), or neutral sign (0) based on the following characteristics.

POSITIVE SUPPORT (+)

- Doesn't eat tempting foods in your presence

- Helps you avoid food you find tempting

- Suggests activities other than eating

- Is interested in and encourages you to meet your goals

- Praises you for your non-weight-related strengths and gifts such as intelligence and creativity

- Helps you brainstorm solutions to your high-risk eating situations

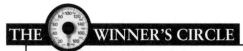

THE WINNER'S CIRCLE

"THE FACT THAT I NEED SUPPORT IS MY FIRST TOOL"

Matti Feldman is currently in her 128th consecutive week of keeping food records.

"I like data, and I find mine interesting to look at," says the 58-year-old Manhattan psychologist, who lost 85 pounds in 1 year.

Interesting yes. But also necessary.

"It's so easy not to make my maintenance my number-one priority," says Feldman. "Keeping food records is one of the ways I keep myself focused."

While recording her food intake is Feldman's primary tool, it's by no means her only one. That's because she's also come to understand her eating patterns and behaviors and has amassed tools to master them.

For example, Feldman isn't a binge-type overeater. "I've learned that I'm a small eater but that I'm quite happy to eat every hour," she says. "For example, I'd be satisfied with one slice of cake. But an hour later, I might like another slice. And 12 hours later, 12 slices are gone."

To keep from nibbling 24/7, Feldman first keeps goodies out of sight, so they're out of mind.

NEGATIVE SUPPORT (−)

- Overeats in front of you
- Tempts you with food
- Encourages you to break your diet or skip the gym "just this once"
- Is critical of your food choices
- Is critical of your appearance

NEUTRAL SUPPORT (0)

- Never discusses weight, yours or anyone else's
- Lets you choose whether or not to eat, without comment

"My husband loves food, and he's a heavy man," she says. "If the treats aren't kept on the counter, I won't root around for them."

When dining out, she often goes halfsies on a main course. "And I never eat a dessert by myself," says Feldman. "I'll share it with my husband or daughter."

Finally, more often than not, she portions out her meals using a food scale and measuring cups and spoons.

Feldman also has a tool that allows her to indulge in her love for fine European chocolate. "I'll portion out and eat one 100-calorie serving—and savor it," she says.

Feldman is as committed to exercise as she is to curbing her nibbling. She wears a pedometer. "Always," she says. "And I walk a lot—at least 5 miles a day, sometimes 10 if I'm not working. I also have a walking partner—my daughter."

But no matter what tools she's using, Feldman is always conscious of the fact that she needs support to keep her program on track.

"It's okay for me to need help," she says. "Maintenance is not something I have to do on my own. It's not something I *can* do on my own. For me, the fact that I need support is the first tool."

- Doesn't try to control your food choices
- Listens when you talk about your problems
- Doesn't give you advice unless you ask for it

EAT #6

Are You Self-Supporting?

WHILE forming a strong social support system is vital, it's equally important to seek other forms of help that you generate on your own. Could you benefit from additional aid and comfort outside of what you receive from family and friends? This portion of the EAT asks you to consider the status of your other self-help outlets.

I use the following support techniques.

	WEEKLY	PERIODICALLY	NEVER
Therapy/counseling sessions	_____	_____	_____
Educational classes in cooking, painting, Italian, or other interest	_____	_____	_____
TOPS, Weight Watchers, or other support group	_____	_____	_____
Stress-reducing techniques such as meditation, yoga, or progressive relaxation	_____	_____	_____
Bodywork classes: tai chi, Alexander technique, or other	_____	_____	_____
Volunteer work	_____	_____	_____
Other	_____	_____	_____

EAT #7

How Active Are You?

THE more you move, the more likely you are to shed pounds or to keep off the pounds you've lost. In fact, members of the National Weight

Control Registry, a group whose members have each lost at least 30 pounds and maintained that loss for at least 1 year, report burning 400 calories in physical activity a day on average. But every little bit of movement helps. In this portion of the EAT, you'll rate your activity level ("activity" meaning both regular workouts and everyday activity) and brainstorm ways to incorporate more movement into your everyday life.

1a. I do the following aerobic activities.

	TIMES/WEEK	DURATION
Aerobic classes/videos	_____	_____
Walking	_____	_____
Jogging	_____	_____
Cycling	_____	_____
Treadmill or elliptical trainer	_____	_____
Other	_____	_____

1b. I do weight training:

Times/Week: _____

Duration: _____

2. Check all of the following that apply.

_____ Whenever possible, I take the stairs instead of the elevator.

_____ When I'm running errands, I park in the far end of the lot and walk to my destination.

_____ I get up to change the channel instead of using the remote.

_____ I open the garage door myself instead of using the automatic opener.

_____ I stand rather than sit when talking on the phone.

_____ I make it a point to take "active breaks" at work (to stroll around the building or the office, walk up and down a flight of stairs, or personally deliver a message rather than e-mail it).

_____ Instead of delivering all of my faxes at the same time, I deliver them one at a time.

_____ I walk to a nearby convenience store for single items instead of hopping into the car.

_____ I park my car at the bottom of a hill and walk up.

Other ways that I can increase my everyday activity:

_____

_____

_____

_____

3. Short-term goal—specific ways that I plan to make my everyday life more active:

_____

_____

_____

_____

_____

4. Long-term goal—specific ways that I plan to make my everyday life more active:

_____

_____

_____

In the next chapter, I'll help you discover what your EAT reveals about your unique eating patterns and behavior. I'll also help you pin down your personal Diet Danger Zones. Even more important, I'll show you how to develop the weight-control strategy that's right for you, based on your unique habits, needs, and lifestyle. As you build your customized plan, you'll decide the best ways to defeat your hidden fat traps, silence your saboteur, build your support system, rev up your physical activity, and more. You'll also devise your Beginner's Tool Kit—but more on that later.

So turn the page and be on your way!

What Your **EAT** Reveals

Now that you've completed your EAT, we can move on to the next phase: developing your customized weight-control plan.

In this chapter, we'll deconstruct your entire EAT. Together, we'll explore what your answers in the preceding chapter reveal about your unique eating and exercise patterns and behaviors. I'll also help you identify your likely Diet Danger Zones and refer you to specific tools in part 2 that may help you master them.

At the end of this chapter, *you* will complete the "Putting It All Together" section, which is the template for your personal weight-control "prescription."

While the assessments you're about to read aren't scientific, they *are* based on my experience helping thousands of clients lose weight and keep it off. Most likely, things you already knew about your overeating will be confirmed here, while you'll be surprised—sometimes even amazed—at what you didn't know.

At this point, I must put in another plug for food journals. If you haven't already read The Ultimate Weight-Loss Weapon: A Pen (page 203), please do. Keeping a journal will help reinforce what you learn about your eating style in this chapter, increasing your odds of success.

Let's go to it!

EAT **#1**: Your Hidden Fat Traps—Revealed

Question 1a

If your EAT indicates that you often skip one meal per day . . .

You're probably trying to "save" calories so you'll lose weight faster. But in truth, you may be consuming more calories than if you ate three meals a day! Think about it. If you're a breakfast-skipper, are you so ravenous by noon that you wolf an enormous lunch? Or do you skip breakfast and lunch to conserve calories, only to go hog-wild at dinner and on into the evening? No doubt about it, skipping meals to conserve calories is a setup for failure.

But who says you have to eat breakfast at 7:00 or 8:00 A.M. or lunch at noon? It doesn't matter *what* time you eat your meals, as long as you're consuming enough calories at one meal to prevent you from eating everything that's not nailed down later on. I am sure that once you stop skipping meals, you'll find it easier not to overeat.

Tools to Try
Food Tools: 7, 8, 35
Mood Tool: 97
Behavior Tools: 150, 151, 155, 197

If your EAT indicates that you skip meals and load up on snacks . . .

You're most likely downsizing your meals to compensate for the considerable calories you consume as snacks. In fact, I'd venture to say that when it comes to portion size, your snacks are the size of a meal, while your meals are probably the size of snacks.

Your goal is to stabilize your eating pattern—that is, the times of day that you eat. You must start eating true meals again—even if you're worried that you won't cut out your snacking and will gain weight.

Tools to Try
Food Tools: 7, 50
Behavior Tools: 159, 162, 173

If your EAT indicates that you load up on bites, tastes, and nibbles . . .

The obvious answer is, "Stop!" This kind of pick-pick-pick eating is always mindless, usually taste-free, and usually guilt-producing.

To become more conscious of your tendency to pick, keep a food diary. When you methodically record those bites and tastes, you'll likely reduce them dramatically.

Tools to Try

Food Tool: 35. You'll be amazed at how many calories those little nibbles contain!

Behavior Tools: All tools under the "Mindless Eating" heading

Question 1b

If your EAT indicates that you tend to eat more during the weekends than during the week . . .

It's likely that you're "good" during the week because you stick to an eating routine. Perhaps you eat at the same time every day, eat the same breakfast and lunch every day, or exercise every Monday and Wednesday after work.

It's that routine—that *structure*—that helps keep your eating on track. So try to extend your Monday-to-Thursday structure through the weekend. Or create a structure just for the weekend. For example, if you normally sleep later on weekends but find a way to get in your three meals a day anyway, start a different routine: Consider making the weekend a two-meal-a-day structure by sitting down to a healthy brunch and a dinner.

Tools to Try

Food Tools: 11, 12, all tools under the "Tools for Social Occasions" heading

Mood Tools: 82, 89

Behavior Tools: All tools under the "Tools for Social Occasions" and "Night and Weekend Eating" headings

Question 1c

If your EAT indicates that you eat more between breakfast and lunch . . .

I'm betting that either your typical breakfast fare doesn't satisfy you or you're particularly vulnerable to the high-fat, high-calorie offerings at the office coffee cart. Either way, your goal is to eat—or eat enough—to satisfy your physical hunger.

Tools to Try

Food Tools: All tools under the "Breakfast" heading, particularly **10**

If your EAT indicates that you eat more between lunch and dinner . . .

Don't get defensive. Snacking between lunch and dinner is often a very good idea. There's often a long span between lunch and dinner, and it's natural to get hungry. But the hours between lunch and dinner are also ripe for mindless eating, as we seek a break from the drudgeries of the workday.

Your mission is to appease true hunger during this time span by *planning* to snack on healthy, filling fare.

Tools to Try

Food Tools: 37, 38, 49, 50
Move Tool: 133
Behavior Tool: 159

If your EAT indicates that you eat more after dinner . . .

You're probably eating out of boredom or to calm yourself after a stressful day at work. Because this is such a common trouble time, I've included lots of tools to help you navigate this dangerous period of time.

Tools to Try

Food Tools: All tools under the "Night Eating" heading
Mood Tool: 89. It can help you see that you can choose not to eat. It can feel very good to make a conscious decision not to give in to your cravings.
Move Tool: 119
Behavior Tools: 160, all tools under the "Night and Weekend Eating" heading

EAT #2: Your Eating Behaviors—Unmasked

Question 1

If your EAT indicates that you eat mostly at-home meals . . .

Great! Cooking at home, rather than dining out, allows *you* to control what you eat, the ingredients you use, and how much you eat. The downside is that you can make your favorite fat- and calorie-laden dishes, and there's no extra charge to you for more than one serving. The key: Assess whom you're cooking for (just you? your family?) and make adjustments in the ways you cook and eat. Again, changing the habits of a lifetime can be difficult—but it may be less difficult than you think.

Tools to Try

Food Tools: 19, 21, 25, 38, 41, 76, all tools under the "Fruits and Vegetables" heading

Mood Tools: 97, 99

Behavior Tools: All tools under the "Eating at Home" heading, all tools under the "Eating Slowly" heading, **164, 165, 167, 170**

If your EAT indicates that you eat most often in restaurants . . .

It's likely that you find it difficult to keep control: The food has hidden fat, the portions are not up to you, and the menu tends to make everything look great. And if you frequent those large good-time chains, the food is fatty, the portions hefty, and the temptation to say, "What the heck, give me the Nachos Grande!" enormous.

Your aim is to establish your own external controls. And that means asking for half-portions, asking for dressing or sauce on the side, and telling your waitperson how you'd like your food prepared. You have to be an active participant in every restaurant meal you choose, whether you dine at a greasy spoon or a four-star eatery. It's difficult, but it can be done. And more often than not, the restaurant will accommodate you. I have a friend who hates garlic. We can go to a four-star restaurant and the waiter has to assure him that nothing he orders will contain the offending bulb. And you know what? He always gets what he wants!

Tools to Try

Food Tools: 11, 12, 15, all tools under the "Tools for Social Occasions" heading

Mood Tools: 100, 107, 112

Behavior Tools: 150, 169, all tools under the "Tools for Social Occasions" heading

If your EAT indicates that you eat at your desk most often . . .

You probably don't give much thought to what you order. Then, when it arrives, you're probably only dimly aware that you're eating it. Like eating in front of the TV, eating at your desk while you work is distracted eating, which can cause even the most dedicated dieters to eat far more than they'd planned—or even were hungry for.

When you eat, you should *eat*, not read the newspaper, call a new account, or play Tetris on your computer. Also, begin to put the same attention into ordering healthy, low-calorie fare as you do eating mindfully.

Tools to Try

Food Tools: 15, 29, 30, 77, all tools under the "Calories: Cuts You'll Never Notice" heading

Mood Tools: 82, 85, 101

Move Tools: 119, 121

Behavior Tools: 156, 161, 173, 204

If your EAT indicates that you eat take-out food most often . . .

Your life is probably hectic (and whose isn't?). So to make it easier, you opt for quick, easy, tasty (sometimes) food cooked by someone else. Totally understandable but ultimately counterproductive. Because along with the quick and easy, you also get hidden calories and fatty special sauces.

You'd do well to choose takeout that's as healthy as it is quick and easy. And yes, you can find it! Instead of heading to a burger or chicken joint, go to a deli and order a sandwich made with lean meat, no cheese, and lots of veggies. If you're on the run, go to a convenience store and buy a carton of low-fat yogurt and a piece of fruit. Get the idea?

Tools to Try
Food Tools: 11, 12, 13, 36, 75, 76, all tools under the "Calories: Cuts You'll Never Notice" heading
Mood Tool: 85
Behavior Tools: 146, 148, 167, 213

If your EAT indicates that you eat most often in front of the TV . . .

It's my opinion that you should stop. When you eat while watching TV (or reading or surfing the Net), you're engaging in what I call hand-to-mouth behavior. What matters isn't what you eat but the comforting and repetitive action of bringing your hand to your mouth.

Tools to Try
Food Tools: 51, 52, 53, 63
Mood Tools: 85, 101, 112
Behavior Tools: 146, 147, 151, 163, 171, 172

If your EAT indicates that you eat most often while standing up . . .

There's only one tool you need for this one: Sit down! (Eating while standing up is mindless eating. There's no use eating if you're not going to remember that you ate it!)

One more thing: From EAT #1, you should now be able to figure out if you're most likely to eat in the morning, afternoon, after dinner, or late at night. Remember this information: You've just pinpointed your high-risk eating time.

Question 2

If your EAT indicates that you tend to eat more when you drink alcohol . . .

You're treading on thin ice. Alcohol can have a "what the heck" effect on your appetite and on what you choose to order. Before you know it, the wine coolers—not you—are ordering the fettuccine Alfredo instead of the grilled salmon.

Tools to Try

Food Tools: All tools under the "Barhopping, Buffets, Cocktail Parties" heading

Behavior Tools: All tools under the "Barhopping, Parties, and Buffets" heading

If you eat *less* when you drink, try to eat salad with some low-fat protein, such as a chicken Caesar salad, to get the nutrients you need.

If your EAT indicates that you tend to eat more when you're at a restaurant . . .

You may be responding to many restaurants' "Eat, drink, have a good time—you deserve it!" atmosphere, which they work hard to cultivate. If you're a sucker for that good-time feeling, your goal is to minimize the temptations of restaurant dining. How? By making eating out as much like eating in—at home—as you can.

Tools to Try

Food Tools: All tools under the "Restaurant Meals" heading

Mood Tools: 89, 96

Behavior Tools: All tools under the "Restaurant Dining" heading

If your EAT indicates that you eat more at home . . .

Commit to making home eating healthy eating. Start bringing home less bacon and more fresh fruit and veggies. If you don't want to nibble, try using one of those over-the-counter night guards you can get at a pharmacy. Put it in your mouth during the times when you usually nibble. It's hard to eat unless you take it out. If you must nibble, it might as well be on low-calorie, high-fiber fare. Generally speaking, though, it's best to stay out of the kitchen between meals, unless you've planned for a healthy snack.

Tools to Try

Food Tools: All tools under the "Fat Battlers" heading, all tools under the "Fruits and Vegetables" heading, all tools under the "Golden Rules" heading

Behavior Tools: All tools under the "Eating at Home" heading, all tools under the "Mindless Eating" heading, **171, 172**

If your EAT indicates that you tend to eat more if you think someone is watching you . . .

You may be . . . angry. Yes, angry. Your overeating is your way of telling the person to go to blazes without actually telling him. Instead of punishing yourself, express your anger in an appropriate way. You might tell these Howard Cosells that their running commentary on your food selections makes you feel that they're sitting in judgment of you, which makes you rebellious and uncomfortable. You may be surprised: They may be astonished and apologize profusely. But even if they don't, you can come to understand that you don't "show" them by what or how much you eat. You only hurt yourself.

Tools to Try
Mood Tools: 95, 99, 108

If your EAT indicates that you tend to eat *less* when someone is watching you . . .

It's important to come out of the closet and allow others to see you eat. The message you convey is, "I'm eating because I choose to eat, and I'm not ashamed of it."

Tools to Try
Mood Tools: 85, 95, 99, 109, 110

If your EAT indicates that you tend to eat more after you've already overeaten . . .

You're operating in the "what the heck" mode. Which is to say, you feel that since you've already blown it, there's no reason to stop eating now. Ah, but there is: You'll do less caloric damage and feel more in control.

Tools to Try
Food Tools: All tools under the "Tools for High-Risk Times" heading
Mood Tools: 88, 89, 95, 106, 109, 110, 112

EAT #3: Your Eating Profile— Outwit Its Weaknesses

If You're a Baby

Likely Diet Danger Zones: 27, 29, 30, 35

If you picked the Baby profile, your mission—should you choose to accept it—is to start taking responsibility for your overeating episodes. No one can make you eat without your consent, from your partner to well-meaning Aunt Pauline.

That said, there *is* a way to soothe your Inner Baby. And that is to allow her to indulge in her favorite foods—within reason. Part of why Babies overeat is because they crave foods they're not "allowed" to have. But if you allow your Inner Baby to have them, she will coo instead of whine (or worse, have an overeating "tantrum"). These tips can help you tame your Inner Baby.

- If your Baby begs for what everyone else is having—the fried mozzarella sticks, the slice of blueberry pie—let her have it. Then, for your next meal, call on your Grown-Up to balance out that indulgence with a lower-calorie meal. (See the "Calories" sections in the Food Tools chapter for nifty tools to help you stay within your calorie range.)

- If your Baby wants to bring home a treat from the supermarket or convenience store, let her. But be firm: If your Baby brings home a whole cake, she'll eat it. So allow her to buy and enjoy two pieces.

- Just like real kids, food Babies need to learn to live within limits. Fortunately, they can, provided you set limits they can live with. For example, if your Baby screams for ice cream, don't offer her ice milk. Let her buy and enjoy a one-serving portion of the real thing. If she wants pizza, allow her one slice. If you force her to have a salad, she'll pitch a fit and may overeat when she gets home. And when she wheedles for her favorite dish, allow her a half-portion—even if it means *you* have to pay for the full portion.

- Ask your Baby to get specific with her cravings. When she wants something, ask her to tell you *exactly what it is that she wants*. If she says, "Chinese food!" ask her to whittle down that desire to one specific dish. If she doesn't, chances are she'll want "everything" and order more than one dish. It's safer for her to decide that what she *really* craves is the sweet and sour chicken. And while her selection may be high in calories, one dish doesn't contain the calories of three, even if she doesn't eat all of them.

If You're an Ostrich

Likely Diet Danger Zones: 15, 19, 20, 31, 35

If you picked this profile, it was probably with extreme reluctance. Ostriches find it hard enough to face up to a bout of overeating or to step on the scale. Unfortunately, by the time they're ready to take their heads out of the sand, their bottoms could be a few sizes larger.

Ostriches would do well to learn the fine art of compartmentalizing. With this tool, you determine the time during the day when you're most likely to overeat. (Your EAT has already indicated these times, so you're halfway there.) Then, you focus on not overeating just during that time of day, using the tools that work for you. Compartmentalizing makes it easier for Ostriches to stop hiding and take action. Here's more advice for this type.

■ Ostriches need to keep a food diary—a recommendation that most of them will fight tooth and nail. As frightening as it can be to record your food intake, it allows you to really see how your eating patterns and behaviors sabotage your weight-control efforts. (For more information on how to keep a food diary, see The Ultimate Weight-Loss Weapon: A Pen on page 203.) One more thing: Record what you eat at the same time you eat it. Ostriches seem to "forget" to record all those bites and tastes if they wait until the end of the day to journal.

■ If you absolutely can't do a food diary, try eating only portions of controlled foods, such as frozen low-calorie meals, steamed vegetables, or a meal-replacement drink. (If you'd like, have one or two small pieces of fruit as well.) Eating portion-controlled food is similar to using a diary because it helps you to become more aware of what you are putting in your mouth. It's also easy. But eat only preportioned foods that list their calorie count. (No "I dunno" foods allowed!)

■ Make this your mantra: "Every bite counts." It's those nibbles, tastes, and bites that can really add up and do Ostriches in.

■ Don't eat in "alone zones" where you can conveniently forget that you've overeaten. Alone zones include your car and the kitchen after everyone has gone to bed.

■ Face your fears, a little at a time. Get into that dress or suit you've been afraid to try on. Take a deep breath and step on the scale. Look at a few photos of yourself at a recent event, even though you've been avoiding doing so. It's scary, yes. But nothing is as scary as not knowing, and you'll also feel pride that you confronted those fears head-on.

If You're a Restrained Eater

Likely Diet Danger Zones: 8, 26, 39, 40

Because you tend to veer between extreme dieting and extreme overeating, you often feel out of control, which is unlikely to help you stick to a safe weight-control program with lasting results. Eating "like a bird" in front of others gives you the illusion that you're in control, which is shattered when you overeat away from the public eye. Restrained Eaters need to learn to eat in public, to own up to their overeating, and to learn to handle situations in which it's easy to eat alone. These suggestions may help.

■ When you dine out, don't even open the menu. Menus make everything appear tempting and will make you feel deprived—which may propel you to the pantry and refrigerator as soon as you get home. (See the "Calories: Stay within Your Range" section of the Food Tools chapter for tips on assembling 300- and 700-calorie meals that you can order anywhere.)

■ The Visual Scale can be a great help to Restrained Eaters because it can help them decide whether they are truly hungry—and help them clarify their options if they're not. (For more about the scale, see tool 97: Visualize your hunger.) *(continued on page 66)*

"WEIGHT MANAGEMENT IS HARD; TOOLS EVEN OUT THE FIGHT"

Susan Bright, the 51-year-old business manager of the New York University School of Law newspaper, takes tools seriously. Very seriously. So much so that in her 5-plus years of working with Cathy, she's filled whole notebooks with them.

"Over the years, I've tried almost every tool I could find," says the Forest Hills, New York, resident. With the help of many, she has dealt in a vastly improved way with her main food issues: portion control and the propensity to binge.

"Tools work because they can teach you new, healthier behaviors and suggest ways to chip away more consistently at old unhealthy ones," says Bright. "The tools I use really make a difference because I use the ones I like."

Obviously. She was 212 pounds when she first began working with Cathy. Now she's 170 pounds—and gearing up to lose more. Integrating the tools that she enjoys has enabled Bright to maintain this 40-pound weight loss for close to 5 years, although achieving and maintaining a lower weight than this remains her longer-term goal.

Utilizing tools has directly benefited her health. Bright, who has diabetes, has seen her blood-sugar levels approach that of a nondiabetic. "And while I take other diabetes medications, the amount of insulin I need has gone down."

Like many of Cathy's clients, Bright sets food policies to help her navigate the treacherous situations that trigger her desire to overeat. Her Danger Zones include holidays and restaurant dining.

For example, her holiday food policy is to choose one or two "must-have" foods and to allow herself very small portions—a few tablespoons of stuffing, a sliver of pie. She keeps the rest of her meal "pure"—lots of vegetables and protein.

She also snaps photographs of her family at these food-laden events.

"I love taking pictures, and you can't eat while you're doing it," she says.

Bright also credits 6 months of cognitive-behavior therapy with her increased ability to more consistently apply techniques that help her pause and think before she eats.

"This therapy has made me much more aware of issues that are at the heart of my bingeing and comfort eating," she says. "If I walk past a bakery and I want to go in and buy something sweet, I've learned to stop and ask myself, 'What just happened?' If the answer is 'nothing,' I ask, 'What happened this morning? Or last night?'"

Whether her desire to eat is triggered by a disagreement with a friend or a car cutting her off, being able to more appropriately connect her feelings with the underlying personal issues "usually gives me time to take a breath and interrupt those feelings," she says. "I have more of a fighting chance to make a better food decision."

Bright never says never to a tool—even if she's dismissed it for years.

"I used to laugh at the "brush your teeth after dinner" suggestion—the idea being that having a fresh, clean mouth discourages nibbling," says Bright. "I thought it was ridiculous. About a month ago, just out of curiosity, I tried it—and it worked."

Bright's other major tool: exercise. "If I could choose just one tool for keeping weight off, working out would be the one." To her regular daily 35- to 40-minute dates with her NordicTrack, she adds yoga, Pilates, and rides on a regular bicycle on the quiet streets of her neighborhood.

No matter which tool Bright happens to pull out of her arsenal, however, she knows that it's bringing her closer to her primary goal: to live long and well.

"As a diabetic, I know weight management is a life or death issue for me," she says. "I'm having a great time, and I want to live a full span of years. Using these tools doesn't totally level the playing field, but it does help fill in some of the deeper potholes."

■ Because Restrained Eaters can nibble away a whole box or bag of something over the course of a day, separate your snacks—healthy or otherwise—into one-serving portions. This way, you'll know exactly how many servings you're eating.

■ Engage in random acts of self-indulgence. Restrained Eaters are often tightly wound and getting into bed early with a trashy novel, getting a massage, or relaxing in a bubble bath can help them see that eating isn't the only pleasure in life.

If You're a Slow Gainer

Likely Diet Danger Zones: 16, 17, 20, 22, 28, 29

The Slow Gainer is an amalgam of all profiles and saboteurs: part Baby, part Ostrich, part Weekend Eater, with a dash of Victim added to the mix. While a Slow Gainer's behavior includes many good habits (otherwise, you'd be gaining weight quickly rather than slowly), you're likely frustrated because it's not clear what you're doing that's causing you to gain. Usually those extra pound-producing calories come in benign blips over a week: an unexpected blowout meal in a restaurant, a piece of birthday cake at an impromptu office party, a pass by the package of dried figs on the kitchen counter. These suggestions can help banish those "blips."

■ Keep a food diary. Because the Slow Gainers' self-defeating eating patterns and behaviors can be so subtle, it's vital that they record what they eat virtually the moment they swallow it. That means every dried fig, every swipe of frosting, every extra chicken nugget you filch off your child's plate while you're clearing the table.

■ For 2 weeks, don't eat between meals. This behavior will make you more conscious of what you're eating while still allowing you to dine out (which pacifies the Weekend Eater in you).

■ If you're a breakfast eater, vary your breakfast fare. Starting the day with a different meal can help to focus the Slow Gainer, even if her previous breakfasts were healthy and steady.

If You're a Weekend Eater

Likely Diet Danger Zones: 13, 26, 38

If you picked this profile, it probably wasn't a tough decision. You most likely can see that from Monday to Friday afternoon, you eat reasonably well. But the weekend is one big food blowout, from Friday-night appetizers and drinks with colleagues to Sunday brunch. It may be that when it comes to eating, you need structure, and weekdays tend to be more structured than anything-goes weekends. So you might think of ways you could put more routine into your weekends, from rising at the same time every Saturday and Sunday morning and eating breakfast at home to designating one weekend night as your "blowout night" while eating normally for the rest of the weekend. The tips below may also help set you straight.

▪ Each week—perhaps on Thursday night—make a list of your weekend food-related events, from a friend's party to a night at the movies. For each event, list the most high-risk foods and situations you're likely to encounter. Then pick the tools that will help you cope with them. (For ideas, see the "Tools for Social Occasions" sections in the Food Tools and Behavior Tools chapters.)

▪ Separate blowout meals into components. Then decide whether you need to eat each part. If you really want the steak dinner, can you live without the garlic bread and baked potato that accompany it and just have a salad? Or can you share the entrée, potato, and all and have a shrimp cocktail as an appetizer? (The "Restaurant Dining" section in the Behavior Tools chapter offers an arsenal of ways to eat what you love without guilt.)

▪ If Sunday brunch is your weakness, order a dish that features the decadence you crave in measured portions: two poached eggs on an English muffin with hollandaise sauce on the side. Or share a side of pancakes. During your other meals, eat tons of vegetables to counterbalance your brunch blowout.

▪ Here's a commonsense tool: If you're skipping meals during the week, stop! Meal skipping or otherwise eating less-than-filling meals during the week to compensate for overeating on the weekends is a setup.

■ Commit to working out at least once during the weekend. Going to the gym on a Friday after work or a Saturday morning can help you maintain the motivation to eat healthfully, too.

If You're a Bad Fairy/Good Fairy

Likely Diet Danger Zones: 5, 8, 10

Because food gives them as much pain as it does pleasure and because they use food as both a punishment and a reward, Good Fairies/Bad Fairies have to learn to stop categorizing food as either "good" or "bad." Food is food, whether it's a piece of death by chocolate cake or a carrot stick. Once they can see food with an objective eye, they're less likely to use it as a reward—or as a weapon.

■ At some point, try the food-mood journal (on page 211) to see if you can link your mood states with your bouts of overeating. Often, you'll see patterns. Did you overeat the day you got lavish praise from your boss or were presented with a civic award? Remember, Good Fairies/Bad Fairies can find it difficult to accept that they deserve good things to happen to them and can negate their successes with self-destructive eating.

■ Whatever situation triggers your urge to eat, ask yourself, "I'm already happy about this. Will overeating add to my happiness? Or is it more likely to make me feel guilty, thereby taking away my *real* reason for being happy?"

■ If you suspect your overeating is a form of self-punishment, ask yourself, "Might I feel as if I deserve to be punished for having it too good and overeat to punish myself? If I couldn't eat, would I punish myself in a different way?"

■ Call a trusted friend or support person and use her as a living, breathing confessional (or psychoanalyst's couch). Tell her what you're about to eat and whether you think you're using this particular food to reward or punish yourself. She may be able to give you some insights into your own behavior.

If You're a Stress Eater

Likely Diet Danger Zones: 2, 4, 5, 7, 8

Stress Eaters tend to "pop" food to calm themselves like other folks pop aspirin to relieve a headache. It doesn't even matter very much what kind of food they eat. (I have known Stress Eaters who have eaten dry Jell-O powder in the throes of a stress-induced eating episode if there was nothing else available.) The mission for Stress Eaters is to teach themselves to relax. But before they can, they must believe that it's within their power to control their stress levels. Try the suggestions below.

▪ Commit to learning at least one simple-to-use stress-relieving technique. Then commit to using it at least once a day for 10 to 15 minutes a day. Many stress-relief books on the market offer step-by-step instruction for meditation, deep breathing, progressive relaxation, along with other stress-relief strategies. To give just two examples: *Mastering Stress 2001: A Lifestyle Approach* by David Barlow and Ronald Rapee and *The Relaxation and Stress Reduction Workbook* by Martha Davis, Elizabeth Eshelman, and Matthew McKay.

▪ If you *must* eat to calm yourself, do it. But make a rule: *You will do nothing else while you stress eat.* You will not watch TV, read, surf the Net, or talk on the phone to a friend. You will focus entirely on your eating. You'll be more aware that you're eating in response to stress, which may help you stop and try one of your stress-busting techniques.

▪ Turn to the "Tools for High-Risk Situations" section of the Mood Tools chapter for more tools that can nip stress eating in the bud.

EAT #4: Your Inner Saboteur—Defanged

If You're a Traditionalist

Face it: You hate change. You cling desperately to the familiar. And when it comes to weight loss, you have your own ideas, thanks—ideas that may be so untrue or out-of-date that they're holding you back!

There are two strains of Traditionalists. The first must take the baby-step approach to change. Try adding food instead of always taking it away. If a vegetable hasn't passed your lips in years, you might make this one small change: Have one vegetable for dinner each night. Other small changes include drinking more water, replacing one specific type of treat (say, doughnut holes) with a piece of fruit or eating an English muffin instead of your usual corn muffin for breakfast.

The second type of Traditionalist needs to dive into change as if she were diving into icy water. For example, she might replace processed foods such as white bread and white rice with whole grain breads, cereals, and brown rice or give up full-fat milk, cream, and cheese for the low-fat or fat-free varieties or give up meat and poultry for vegetarian fare.

Whichever Traditionalist you are, your goal is to take some kind of action, no matter how small. Pushing yourself to try one new behavior will spur you to try others. And the positive changes that result from those behaviors will make it easier to make more changes.

If You're a Perfectionist

The Navajo Indians say that every blanket they make contains a slight imperfection because only God is perfect. If you're a Perfectionist, you'd do well to take this lesson to heart. Your weight-control efforts will go much more smoothly—and are likely to be more successful—if you accept that you *will* have lapses and that there's no need to atone for them by overeating (and then starving yourself the next day).

Here's a visual scale tailor-made for Perfectionists. Draw this:

Failure ——————————————————————————————Perfection

Find a point on the continuum that correlates to how you currently feel about your weight-control efforts. Perfect, because you followed your plan to the letter? Like a failure, because you ate half the fries from your child's Happy Meal? Somewhere in between? Place an X at that point. Ideally, your X would be somewhere between the middle and perfection, indicating that you feel neither like a saint nor a failure. (See also tool 95: Challenge your beliefs about perfection.)

If You're a Rebel

To tame the "who's gonna stop me?" side of you, try including so-called forbidden foods as part of a meal and substantially reduce the calories in the remainder of the meal.

Make a list of the things you want: cake, steak, ice cream, nachos dripping with cheese, a jumbo bag of M&M's. Now, have one of them in one-serving increments—at every meal, if you wish. The rest of your meal is steamed vegetables or a salad with low-fat or fat-free dressing on the side. For example, if you crave a steak, have it—along with your large salad. Or have a salad and two slices of chocolate cake. Or a double scoop of ice cream with, yes, a salad. Or a giant corn muffin and a salad. Take heed: If your portions of vegetables or salads shrink while those of your "fun foods" grow larger, this tool doesn't work for you.

This isn't the most nutritious way to eat, and you can't eat this way forever—only when you're feeling particularly surly about what you think you can and can't have. Don't eat this way for more than 2 weeks at a time and take a good daily multivitamin.

If You're a Victim

As difficult as it is for you to assert yourself, learning to do so is the only way to break free from the grips of this saboteur. What this means is that you gather the courage to order the healthy, low-calorie meal *you* want, regardless of what your partner, a friend, or a business client orders. Tell a friend who's throwing a party that you'd like to bring raw veggies and dip or a fruit salad, so you'll have something to nosh other than chips. Call your mother before you arrive for Thanksgiving dinner, tell her you'll be bringing your own meal (or eating only the low-calorie offering on her table), and ask that she not push food on you.

I realize that Victims find it extremely uncomfortable to express their needs and to ask for what they want. The following exercise can help you find the road to assertiveness.

Divide a piece of paper into four columns. In the first column, list possible situations in which you might feel like a "food victim" (at a family dinner, with a food-pushing best friend, at a business lunch, and so on). In the second column, make a list of options. What could you do other than go along with what everyone else is eating or cave in to the pressure to eat? After you list those options, try one or all of them. In the third column, list the options you tried and which ones worked. In the last column, list the options that didn't work and why.

Take another look at column three. Know what you just did? You wrote your own tools. Now, go forth and conquer!

EAT #5: Your Support System: How Strong Is It?

You can't always choose your family and coworkers. But you *can* keep anyone who sabotages your weight-control efforts at arm's length and learn to ask for help from those who would gladly offer their support.

Look at the diagram you drew in your EAT, noting the position of the positive, negative, and neutral folks in your life.

To Attract Positives

At work: Try to bring them closer. Drop into their office for moral support before or after you must deal with a negative colleague. Ask if they'd like to join you in an after-lunch walk. In the cafeteria, ask if you might join them. Of course, don't be pushy or intrusive. But if you feel that you can trust them, do let them know that you enjoy their company and could use their support.

Long-distance friends and relatives: Make a commitment to call and e-mail more often. If one of these folks wants to lose a few pounds as well, you could launch your own mini-support group. E-mail them every day to report on your progress. Share tools that have worked for you and ask them for their most helpful tools.

Immediate family or friends: Ask for their support when you know you'll be confronting one of your Diet Danger Zones.

I once had a client who went to a family reunion that her mother, who lived in another state, was hosting. Her mother was a food pusher, and my client knew she would exhort her to eat. So she told her siblings that she was on an all-formula diet and asked them to help her stand up to her mother.

They did, and she did. She stayed on the formula and lost weight, and everyone had a good time—even Mom!

To Neutralize Negatives

At work: These are the colleagues who urge you to splurge when the group goes out to lunch, the coworker who keeps an eagle eye on your weight-loss progress and feels free to comment on your food choices, or anyone who keeps a stash of high-fat, high-calorie snacks on his desk. To keep your distance, perhaps you can eat lunch earlier or later, lunch with your colleagues only when that person won't be joining you, or take the long way to the copy or fax machine so you won't have to pass that person's office.

Family members who don't live with you: Call rather than visit. Or if you must visit—say, you have a standing Sunday-afternoon dinner at their place—bring your own dinner and snacks. You might even eat before you go, so you don't have room for more than a salad and a cup of coffee. (Let them raise their eyebrows or make a snide remark. Let it go: Realize that they are used to your "old" self and that you have to help them understand the new you.)

Family negatives who live with you: If you can't convert them to your cause, protect yourself. See the prescriptions in Diet Danger Zones 13, 14, 22, 32, 34, and 40.

To Scope Out the Neutrals

Your diagram may include some "neutrals"—people who aren't clearly positives or negatives. Observe them for a while. What does your gut say? Follow your instincts. If a particular neutral seems well-meaning but triggers distrust in you, place her in the negative category. (You won't hurt her feelings. She doesn't have to know.)

If, however, you decide a neutral could be a force for good, take her aside. Without embarrassment or making a big deal out of it, explain that you're trying to lose weight and ask her if she's willing to lend her support. If she is, be prepared to tell her—friend, family member, or colleague—exactly what she can do to help.

One more thing: As your life changes, so might your support system. So take EAT #5 several times a year to see if it's changed. If it has, update it.

EAT #6: Self-Support: Can You Be There for You?

Whether you're in the weight-loss phase or trying to maintain your new, lighter weight, it's crucial to learn to be a source of support to *yourself*. After all, successful weight loss is a by-product of self-love and self-esteem. The more you have, the more successful you're likely to be.

How many sources of self-generated support were you able to list?

■ 0–1 source of support: **Suss out some support.** Now is the time to discover or resume an interest or hobby that fascinated you in the past or to open yourself to something entirely new.

You may just find that being there for yourself and focusing on the care and feeding of your mind and soul can help keep you from "eating yourself up."

■ 2–4 sources of support: **You're doing great!**

Whether you've started therapy, are taking a class, or are doing volunteer work, you're able to reach out. And the more you can give to others, the more you can give to *you*.

■ 5–7 sources of support: **Congratulations!**

It's likely that you're one of your own best friends and have the ability to comfort yourself. Just as important, you can focus on the world around you, instead of just on the numbers on your scale.

EAT #7: Are You Moving Enough?

Question 1a

If your EAT indicates that you get less than 30 minutes of aerobic exercise at least three times a week . . .

You're not meeting the recommended standards for aerobic exercise set by the government. *Please* don't feel discouraged or guilty about that. Starting and sticking to a regular exercise program can be tough. The key is to commit to doing as much as you can and to do it consistently. Even committing to 10 minutes of brisk walking twice a week is a start.

Once you feel comfortable with that, try setting short- and long-term exercise goals. Start an activity diary. The goal would be twofold: to try to be consistent with your exercise (even if it's a little bit) and to try to do it more often.

To learn how to set realistic goals, see tool 88: Go for the goals.

Question 1b

If your EAT indicates that you get less than 20 minutes of weight training twice a week . . .

See the suggestions above. Doing some form of resistance training twice a week for 20 minutes is all it takes to get and stay toned, firm, and strong. And there's good reason to make this tiny time investment. Lifting does more than give you shapelier muscles and change your proportion of muscle to fat, which helps you burn more calories. It also helps keep your bones strong and fracture-free and gives you more energy. For ways to get started, see tool 130: Put up some resistance.

Question 2

If your EAT indicates that you do five or more of the everyday activities listed . . .

Keep it up! If less than five, keep working at it. The more you move, the easier it will be to move more. See the Move Tools chapter for ways to incorporate more movement into your daily life.

Questions 3 and 4

I asked you these questions so that you could begin to set some get-moving goals for yourself. Take a close look at what you've written. Are your goals realistic, specific, and achievable? For help in formulating fitness goals, see tool 88: Go for the goals.

Putting It All Together

Hopefully, you're now more aware of the ways in which your unique eating and exercise patterns and behavior help—and hurt—your weight-loss or maintenance program. Perhaps you've found that you snack more than you thought. Or that you need more of a social support network. Or that you eat well at home but blow it when you dine out.

Whatever you've learned, now's the time to pull it all together.

Photocopy this page and pages 77 and 78. Then, using the space provided, answer the following questions as honestly as you can. Since you've not yet become intimately acquainted with the tools or your Diet Danger Zones, fill out as much as you can and guess about the rest. (Your guesses might point you in the right direction!)

After you're more familiar with the tools and have identified your Diet Danger Zones, retake this quiz. In fact, come back to this quiz whenever you feel that your eating or exercise programs are adrift or take it on a quarterly basis to keep yourself motivated to continue your program.

1. List three things that are working especially well in your program. Examples: You're working out three times a week consistently; you've cut way down on your nighttime eating; at home, you eat only at the dining-room table.

_____

_____

_____

2. List the eating or exercise program you might try if the one you're using now doesn't work. Examples: a high-fiber diet, cutting back on carbohydrates, eating only portion-controlled meals such as frozen diet entrées.

_____

_____

_____

3. List three ways that you could improve one aspect of your eating or exercise program right now. Be as specific as you can. (Stumped? Take a look through your EAT for ideas.)

_____

_____

_____

4. List what you still need to learn to help you succeed with your weight-loss or maintenance program. Examples: to avoid wandering into the kitchen after dinner, to make time for a healthy breakfast at home rather than stopping at a fast-food drive-thru.

_____

_____

_____

5. List three things that you can do right now to get the support you need. Examples: asking a friend or your partner for help in following your program and telling him exactly how he can help, signing up for a water-aerobics class at the Y.

_____

_____

_____

6. List the specific times, meals, or situations (if any) when you are comfortable with eating—when you feel strong and in control. Examples: breakfast, after 9:00 P.M. on weeknights (perhaps you're

going to bed earlier), when people try to foist food that you don't want on you (you've learned to say, "No, thank you").

_____

_____

_____

7. List the specific times or situations (if any) when your eating tends to get out of control. Examples: being at home alone, at a restaurant, on weekends, at night.

_____

_____

_____

8. List your most important short-term goal.

_____

_____

_____

9. List your most important long-term goal.

_____

_____

_____

10. List any other comments, questions, or concerns that you may have about weight loss and your unique approach to it. You may not have the answers now, but hang in there. If you do the work, the answers will be revealed.

_____

_____

_____

Part 2

THE TOOLS: MORE THAN 200 WAYS TO OUTWIT YOUR WEIGHT

Learn the Tool Basics

Many overweight people know a lot about food and nutrition. They can debate the nutritional pros and cons of any diet plan and rattle off, to the half-calorie, the calorie content of a cup of pasta or a banana. But few can translate what they know about weight loss into *action*. And knowledge without action is useless.

That's where tools come in. They show you how to turn what you know about eating and exercise into a concrete action plan for success.

Before you dive into the tools, understand that many different tools can be used to master the same situation or challenge. So if you don't like one tool, you're free to try another.

Say you tend to gobble your food. You know eating more slowly can help you avoid overeating, but you frequently forget to do it. To translate what you *know* to do into *action*, you can try any of a number of tools that address this specific challenge. You can divide the food on your plate in half and take a 10-minute break at "halftime." Or you can use chopsticks to remind you of the importance of eating slowly. And those tools are just for starters.

Also, be aware that tools aren't "one size fits all." A tool that's right for you may be wrong for your mother, sister, or colleague. Elsewhere in this book, I suggest tools that may be right for you, based on your unique characteristics and Diet Danger Zones.

But ultimately, to know if a tool will work for you, you have to try it. Choosing and using tools is a matter of try, try again, but it's amazing how quickly you can amass an arsenal of tools that work for you.

You already know what it takes to lose weight. Tools can help you actually *do it*, regardless of what diet you're on. As you become more familiar with choosing and using tools, you'll come to see that there's no situation you can't handle, no challenge you can't master . . . as long as your tool kit is full.

The Food Tools

Everyday Tools: Slimming Strategies to Live By

BREAD: CONTROL YOUR CRAVINGS

1. Follow the rule of two.

Don't eat more than 2 ounces of bread at a time. One slice of sandwich bread is about 1 ounce, a small roll is about 2 ounces, a sandwich roll is 3 to 4 ounces, a bagel is 4 to 6 ounces. Yes, that means you should eat half a bagel or half a sandwich roll at a time.

2. Eat bread when it counts.

One way is to limit yourself to no more than 2 ounces at every meal. Or have bread once a day, at the meal you enjoy it most. For example, if you like bread best at lunch, don't have a bagel for breakfast. You'll waste your bread allotment.

3. Knock bread off the dinner menu.

Sometimes, it's easier to avoid a problem food than it is to eat it in moderation. So if you love to have bread at dinner but tend to eat too much of it, don't have bread at this meal. End of story. You'll eventually think "I never have bread at dinner" rather than "I _can't_ have bread at dinner."

4. Go with the (whole) grain.

Eat only whole grain bread. It's more nutritious than white bread. It's also harder to find, which helps you to think before you reach.

Note that a pumpernickel bagel or a bran muffin is more white flour than whole grain. To make sure you choose a bona fide whole grain product, read the label. The first ingredient should say "100 percent whole wheat." If it says "enriched," "unbleached," or "unbromated," it's made with white flour; leave it on the shelf.

5. Resist restaurant bread.

Can't keep your mitts out of the bread basket when you dine out? See tool 74: Master the bread basket.

BREAKFAST: THE ANYTIME MEAL

6. Do breakfast for dinner.

If you tend to overeat at lunch or dinner, consider replacing that meal with healthy breakfast fare. Most of us feel good about how much we eat for breakfast, as we're not likely to have eight slices of toast or six bowls of cereal.

7. Make breakfast a "mini."

If you don't like to eat breakfast first thing in the morning, don't. But if you tend to snack too much between meals, save breakfast for a time when you need a more substantial snack. You might have it as a mini-meal at midmorning or between lunch and dinner.

8. Join the breakfast club.

If you skip breakfast because you think you're saving calories and will lose weight more quickly, think again. Some research suggests that being overweight and skipping breakfast may be related. So if you're hungry in the morning, by all means eat.

9. Make breakfast a morning snack.

If you can't even look at food in the morning but are always so ravenous by lunch that you tend to overeat, you might try to eat something later in the morning—your "morning snack."

Experiment and see how much food you can handle. Perhaps a piece of fruit is enough. Or you might try a cup of instant oatmeal, a slice of whole grain toast spread with a tablespoon of peanut butter, or even a mini turkey sandwich on a small whole wheat pita.

10. Phase out your second breakfast.

If you usually eat two breakfasts—the one you planned at home and the one you inevitably have at the office—consciously choose to eat the one that's harder to give up. That's usually your office breakfast.

If you get hungry at home before you get to work, eat a piece of fruit and save your cereal or whole grain toast for the office. Or if you must have that Danish from the office breakfast cart, enjoy it and count it among your empty calories. If when you go to the breakfast cart to get your morning coffee, the pastry cries out to you, ask a sympathetic colleague to get your coffee.

CALORIES: STAY WITHIN YOUR RANGE

11. Assemble an arsenal of 300-calorie meals.

Make sure they're meals that you can get anywhere, whether you're at home or on the go. Here are a few examples: a meal-replacement drink or bar, a BLT without mayo, poached eggs on a dry English muffin, a bowl of clear soup and a salad with low-fat dressing on the side, a bowl of clear soup and two containers of low-fat yogurt. Use your calorie counter to create others.

12. Follow up with 700-calorie meals.

Whip out your calorie counter and assemble dinners you can order in a diner or at the finest four-star restaurant. Here's one example of a 700-calorie meal: a glass of wine, a shrimp cocktail, some steamed vegetables, a half-portion of pasta with marinara sauce or a broiled chicken breast, and a small baked potato.

13. Try the Chinese-menu plan.

Here's a fun way to preplan your food choices. Arrange the foods you tend to eat most into lists according to the calories they contain. In the following list, column A contains 150-calorie foods; column B, 80-calorie foods; column C, 25-calorie foods; and column D, 60-calorie foods. Mix and match to fit your daily calorie allotment.

For example, for lunch, you might have about 550 calories: 1 food from column A, 3 from column B, 4 from column C, and 1 from column D; or 5 from column B, 4 from column C, and 1 from column D. Write out and photocopy your list so you can carry it with you everywhere.

A (150 calories)	B (80 calories)	C (25 calories)	D (60 calories)
3 oz skinless chicken	3 oz potato	½ cup cooked broccoli	½ grapefruit
8 oz tofu	⅓ cup cooked rice	½ cup cooked mushrooms	1 medium apple
6 oz shellfish	½ cup cooked pasta	4 asparagus spears	1 orange
¾ cup cottage cheese	1 slice bread	½ cup cooked carrots	1 kiwifruit
4 oz tuna	1 ear corn	1 cup greens	2 tangerines
6 oz shrimp	½ cup cooked peas	½ cup cooked cauliflower	1 pear
6 tsp Parmesan	⅓ cup cooked dry beans	½ cup cooked green beans	½ cantaloupe
3 oz flank steak	½ cup cooked yams	½ artichoke	1 cup strawberries
1 cup fat-free yogurt	1 oz cereal	½ cup cooked beets	1 cup watermelon

14. Scale down the big four.

If you tend to overeat on pasta, bread, rice, or potatoes, omit them from your diet. One of my patients used this tool and lost a significant amount of weight. I'm not advocating a low-carbohydrate diet. You'll still be eating cereal, beans, fruits, and vegetables.

15. Don't play dumb with calorie counts.

If you're finding it difficult to lose weight or maintain your desired weight, consider how often you eat "I dunno" foods. These are foods with an unknown number of calories. They include ethnic dishes such as Chinese and Indian food, casseroles, and deli pasta salads.

When you eat "I dunno" foods, you may well consume more calories than you realize. In fact, the *New York Times* evaluated various plain cheese pizzas and found that they ranged from 400 to 900 calories a slice!

Bottom line: If you can't tally its calories, think twice before you eat it.

CALORIES: CUTS YOU'LL NEVER NOTICE

16. Make small changes, save big calories.

Make slight changes in your food choices. This tool can save you tons of calories but still allow you to eat a decent amount of food. A few examples:

■ Instead of 1 cup of creamed corn for 184 calories, eat corn on the cob for 83 calories.

■ Instead of 2½ cups of pasta at 490 calories, have 1 cup of pasta mixed with 1¼ cups of steamed broccoli florets and 1 cup of steamed sliced mushrooms at 265 calories.

■ Instead of an appetizer of five fried mozzarella sticks (500 calories), have 20 small steamed clams (133 calories). Just don't dip them in butter.

■ Instead of 1 cup of granola (500 calories), have 1 cup of oatmeal with half a banana (200 calories).

17. Dodge coffeehouse sabotage.

Get this: A 12-ounce serving of café mocha at one popular coffeehouse chain packs a whopping 340 calories and 21 grams of fat. That's because it's laden with chocolate, warm milk, and whipped cream. To slim down coffeehouse offerings, ask the server to use fat-free milk and hold the whipped cream, heavy cream, chocolate sprinkles, and syrups.

18. Put syrup on the side.

Rather than pour maple syrup all over your pancakes or waffles, measure out a tablespoon and put it in a small dish. Then dip your pancakes or waffles into the dish.

19. Give ground beef a bath.

To reduce the fat in ground beef, brown it, then place it in a colander and douse with boiling water.

20. Cha-cha over to salsa.

At 5 calories a tablespoon, low-fat salsa isn't just for burritos anymore. Use it on baked potatoes and as a topping for sandwiches or vegetables. You can even mix it with fat-free sour cream for a creamy, zesty salad dressing.

21. Top salads with a guilt-free crunch.

Why ruin a perfectly good low-calorie salad with oily croutons? Instead, crush a crumbled-up flavored rice cake and toss onto your greens.

22. Deflate the overstuffed sandwich.

When you order a sandwich—no matter what the filling—ask for half the amount they usually serve.

23. Play hardball with soft drinks.

Cut back or completely eliminate soda from your diet. Or at least consider doing so. There's evidence that our bodies might not register the calories we drink as well as they do the calories we eat. Liquid calories just don't appear to switch off our appetites. Which means that if we regularly drink large quantities of soda (or other high-calorie drinks), we might not eat less food to compensate.

Consider this study: Researchers asked people to consume 450 calories' worth of jelly beans a day for 4 weeks and 450 calories' worth of soda a day for another 4 weeks. On jelly-bean days, these folks ate roughly 450 fewer calories, consuming no more calories than usual. But on soda days, they ate about 450 *more* calories than usual!

To cut back . . .

- Order a small or child-size soda instead of a large or super-size serving.

- Ask for lots of ice in your soda if you order it in a cup. You get less soda and fewer calories.

- Get an extra cup and split a soda with a friend. If the waiter offers a free refill, ask for water.

24. Dilute fruit juice with water.

If you love fruit juice, beware. Depending on the serving size, you could be swallowing hundreds of calories (especially if you buy those 20-ounce bottles). To shave extra calories, dilute juice by half with water or seltzer. Or better yet, forgo the juice and have the real thing: fruit.

25. Don't "eyeball" oil.

Whether you drizzle your salad with olive oil or stir-fry your veggies with canola oil, measure it. Always. That quarter cup of oil you drizzle into the frying pan packs a hefty 482 calories. And if you don't measure it out, you're bound to add a whole lot more.

FAT BATTLERS: FOODS THAT FIGHT FAT

26. Block fat with calcium.

If your diet plan allows low-fat dairy products, don't skimp on them. A preliminary study suggests that people who take in the most calcium from food (about 1,300 milligrams a day) reduce their chances of becoming overweight by a whopping 80 percent compared with those who take in only 255 milligrams daily. In another study, researchers at the University of Tennessee in Knoxville found that mice getting the most calcium stored less fat than those consuming less calcium.

Whether calcium really helps humans stay leaner remains to be seen. But there's no harm in upping your intake of this important mineral. So drink up! Try this thick shake as a snack: Blend 8 ounces of fat-free milk with a frozen banana, some ice, and 1 teaspoon of vanilla extract until smooth. Absolutely delicious!

27. Boost your fiber quota.

Consuming lots of fruits, vegetables, and whole grains helps you eat less because these plant-based foods contain a large amount of fill-you-up fiber. Experts estimate that each gram of fiber substituted for simple carbohydrates such as sugary foods results in a loss of 7 calories. So if you double your daily fiber intake from 10 or 15 grams—the amount the average American consumes—to 26 grams, you'd save yourself an average of 100 calories!

FRUITS AND VEGETABLES: MORE FOOD FOR FEWER CALORIES

28. Reconfigure your plate-to-produce ratio.

If you hate to count calories, follow the "plate rule." Visualize half your plate filled with vegetables and the other 50 percent divided between meat and starch. If you're in a restaurant, follow the plate rule by ordering an extra dish of steamed vegetables and sharing your chicken with a friend. Or order a half-portion of pasta and an extra plate of steamed vegetables and combine the two.

29. Factor in produce first.

Preplanning your food day can put portion size and healthy eating into better perspective. Another way to plan your food day is to include vegetables first. They're nutritious and filling, yet tend to be overlooked.

Then add fruit and small portions of high-fiber starches, such as brown rice, whole grain bread, and beans. To achieve peak nutrition, add a high-calcium food like yogurt or an ounce of reduced-fat cheese. Finally, add high-protein foods, such as fish, chicken, and meat.

Note that there's hardly any room left in your food day for fat and sugar. Which means, of course, that you'll eat them in very small quantities!

30. Color-code your plate.

Think of fruits and vegetables as a box of colorful crayons and play with color combinations. Pair the rich purple hue of eggplant with the sunny

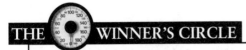
THE WINNER'S CIRCLE

"MY MAIN TOOL? PLANNING MEALS THAT WORK AND WILL SATISFY ME"

For attorney Amy Guss, maintaining her 25-pound weight loss boils down to a simple, yet critical, formula: Three parts careful food planning plus one part regular exercise.

"The main tool I use is planning meals that work and will satisfy me," says Guss, who's maintained her weight loss for more than 2 years. "I have two or three meal options I can choose from for breakfast, and maybe three or four options to choose from for lunch. That can really help you stay on track."

For breakfast, Guss chooses yogurt and fruit or a single serving of pre-packaged cold cereal with fruit. On cold winter days, she opts for single-serving portions of oatmeal. Her lunch options include healthy salads of chicken or tuna combined with olive oil, and vegetable salads made with broccoli or other healthy, vitamin-rich unrefined carbohydrates. "One option when you're particularly hungry and know salad at lunch isn't going to do it is a turkey sandwich on whole wheat," Guss says.

Dinner options include light fare such as a veggie burger or soup and a small, low-calorie frozen entrée. Greek salads with feta cheese are also part of Guss's dinner repertoire.

At lunch and dinner, Guss follows Cathy's advice to fill two-thirds of her

orange of peppers or cantaloupe. Combine the deep emerald green of collard greens with the rich red of strawberries for dessert. Your plate will be as gorgeous as it is nutritious.

31. Flirt with vegetarianism.

Sometimes, consciously trying to eat in a new way makes it easier to eat less. So experiment with a meatless menu for a few days or even a week and see if you like it. Try stir-fried tofu, soy burgers or franks, or vegetable stew.

A word to the wise: Watch the full-fat dairy products. Cheese, in par-

plate with vegetables, leaving the remaining one-third for low-fat forms of protein such as chicken or fish. Guss also limits refined carbohydrates such as bread. "I don't totally stay away from carbs, but I do keep them down," she says.

Yet when it comes to exercise, Guss's attitude is "The more the merrier." "I pretty much spend most of my time at work sitting," says Guss. "There's no way around it: I must work out four to five times a week."

Knowing life can stall even the best-laid plans for exercising, Guss is a big believer in flexibility. If the weather's good, she runs outside. If she can't get to the park, she jogs at the gym. And if running isn't an option, she'll walk to work or sweat it out on her health club's elliptical trainer.

After a long day, Guss reaches into her tool bag to satisfy her sweet tooth: She plans specific treats such as a small bowl of mango ice with blueberries, which provide the sugar she craves but won't leave her vulnerable to overeating. "Plan a treat you know you'll be able to handle," she advises. "I would not plan to have a chocolate chip cookie at night," she says. "But mango ice? That, I can handle. It's refreshing, and it cleanses the palate."

ticular, is laden with fat and calories. Opt for low-fat or fat-free milk, cheese, and yogurt.

32. Stock up on frozen veggies.

If the fresh vegetables you buy tend to rot in the crisper before you get around to preparing them, buy frozen vegetables instead. Whether you toss them into stir-fries or pasta, they're full of fiber and nutrients, they'll help fill you up, and they'll reduce the amount of pasta or rice you eat. Put them in your favorite soup or pasta sauce, mix them with brown rice, or pile them on burritos.

33. Go on a vegetable safari.

Each week, prowl the produce aisle and select a vegetable you've either never tried or tried once and disliked. Then find out how to cook it in a low-fat, low-calorie manner. (There are often recipe ideas for veggies nearby. Or you can surf the Internet for recipes.) This tool offers you the perfect opportunity to expose yourself or your vegetable-shy family to exotic alternatives like bok choy, collard or mustard greens, and artichokes. You can go on safaris for exotic fruits and spices, too.

GOLDEN RULES: 10 TOOLS TO LIVE BY

34. Cut 250 calories a day.

Once you've determined your optimal calorie level, shave 250 calories from your daily total. You'd be surprised where you can find these calories—that extra half-cup of breakfast cereal, the rice cakes in the afternoon, that trip into the kitchen after dinner for a cup of tea and "a little something." With this simple tool alone, you can drop 25 pounds in a year!

35. Tally "tastes."

Always record tastes in your food diary. A spoonful of this or a fingerful of that may not register in your brain as eating, but it is. Here's how many calories you consume when you "taste" about 1 tablespoon of the following foods.

Cake icing: 55

Cream cheese: 50

Gravy: 40

Leftovers on your partner's or child's plate: 50–100

Maple syrup: 52

Nuts: 50

Peanut butter: 100

Raisins: 30

Salad dressing: 40

Sour cream: 30

Surprised? Good. Chances are you'll think twice before you pop a few olives into your mouth or eat just the icing off a slice of a colleague's birthday cake.

36. Learn to eyeball portions.

When you're out in public and can't whip out the measuring cups, it's essential to know how to guesstimate portion sizes. Here's what real servings of common foods look like.

- 1 cup breakfast cereal: the size of a baseball
- 3 ounces meat: a regular-size bar of soap
- 3 ounces hamburger: fits in a mayonnaise-jar lid
- 1 cup pasta (2 ounces dry): a Walkman
- 1 ounce cheese: a Ping-Pong ball
- 2 tablespoons peanut butter: a large walnut in the shell
- 1 ounce potato chips or pretzels: fits in both your open, cupped palms
- 1 ounce nuts: fits in one cupped palm
- 1 teaspoon butter: the tip of your thumb
- 2 tablespoons salad dressing: a full shot glass
- 1 slice of pie: 4 knuckles' worth (1 knuckle's worth equals 100 calories)

37. Water tool 1: Get in the drink.

Like plants, humans need water. But H_2O does more than just ensure our survival. Drinking at least 10 to 12 glasses (8 ounces) of liquid a day—making 5 of them plain water—can make us feel fuller and enhance our health. If you're more camel than human and hate to drink water, take heart: Getting those 40 ounces is simpler than you think. At work, keep a full 20-ounce water bottle on your desk and drink until it's empty. Keep an identical water bottle at home and drain it dry before you turn in.

38. Water tool 2: Sip, bite, sip, bite . . .

Divide your meal in half. At the halfway mark, drink a glass of water. It will slow your eating, help you meet your water quota, and maybe even fill you up a little more.

39. Never eat from the source.

See tool 171 in the Behavior Tools chapter.

40. Don't play the "it doesn't count if . . ." game.

This tool is similar to tool 35, but it's especially helpful for those of us who tend to sample other people's entrées in a restaurant.

Just as you record those couple of spoonfuls of peanut butter in your food diary, record that forkful of pasta primavera and that shared slice of tiramisu. Even if you don't know how many calories each forkful or spoonful contains, you'll know to forgo dessert or a second glass of wine.

41. Chew gum while you cook.

See tool 210 in the Behavior Tools chapter.

42. Overindulged? Use the day-after tactic.

The day after you overeat, return to your weight-loss or maintenance plan. But for this one day, cut 200 to 500 calories from your daily calorie allotment. Or burn off some of those extra calories with exercise. (Fun fact: If she walks 3 miles an hour, a 200-pound woman can burn off a slice of apple pie in 78 minutes.)

43. Cook when you're least likely to eat.

If you have to make potato salad for the picnic, bake cookies for the school-board meeting, or prep for your dinner party, try to do it at the time when you eat the least. (For most people, that's morning.)

HUNGER BLOCKERS: TOOLS TO TAME A RAGING APPETITE

44. Eat less, more often.

If you're usually ravenous by the time your next meal rolls around, break up your meals. For example, if you typically eat a bowl of soup and a sandwich for lunch, have your sandwich at lunchtime and your soup 2 hours later. Do the same with your dinnertime salad or potato.

45. Or eat more, less often.

If you prefer to eat just three times a day with no between-meal noshing, have larger meals, making sure you stay within your allotted calorie amount. Center your meals around high-protein, low-fat foods—such as poached eggs, fish, and lean meats—and include plenty of vegetables to fill you up.

46. Start low, end high.

Look at your plate. Pick out the lowest-calorie food (typically, your veggies). Eat the vegetables first to fill you up. Then eat the next-lowest-calorie item. Save your highest-calorie item for last. You may be too full to finish it.

47. Or start high, end low.

If you tend to keep eating because you left your favorite food for last, eat the foods you like best first so you have less room for calories you don't care about.

My hope is that you'll also have room for the most nutritious foods. But if you're going to listen to your hunger, you should stop eating when you feel full, even if you have to leave your steamed broccoli on your plate.

48. Don't forgo dietary fat.

Yes, beef, cheese, and peanut butter are high in fat. But if you like them, don't eliminate these foods entirely. Eating small portions of the "forbidden" foods you love can make the difference between adjusting to healthier eating and rejecting it because you feel that you can't have the foods you love.

Try your eggs poached instead of fried. Buy a tiny amount of fresh-ground peanut butter instead of a whole jar, which tempts you to eat more than one serving. Treat yourself to an ice cream cone rather than bring a half-gallon of your favorite flavor into the house.

49. Identify your prime snack time.

Most of us snack at the same time every day, yet we don't plan it into our food day. Pinpoint that time and plan ahead for what to snack on. For example, if you tend to get hungry right before dinner, plan your snack then. If you have a small snack an hour or so before dinner, you're likely to eat an appropriate amount at that meal. Just *please* don't eat a huge snack and skip dinner. You'll probably feel ravenous later in the evening, increasing your risk of overeating.

50. Stretch your lunch.

If you tend to get hungry in the late afternoon, eat half your lunch at the regular time and the other half as an afternoon snack.

51. Buy single-serving snacks.

Cookies, chips, and even ice cream come in single-serving sizes. If you want them, eat a little bag instead of a whole big box. If you prefer to buy large packages to save money, use sealable plastic bags or storage containers and repackage the food into single-size servings.

52. Keep snacks under wraps.

Now that you buy individual-size snacks, hide these little bags and containers. Put them behind the boxes of rice and pasta in your pantry, so you'll really have to work to dig them out.

53. Opt for eat-slow snacks.

Foods that are hard to eat take longer to finish, which gives your brain a chance to compute what's in your stomach. Some hard-to-eat, easy-to-love snacks include:

- Two large carrots (Dip each bite in salsa.)

- Five low-fat crackers topped with fat-free cream cheese and scallions (Can't eat just five? Make up the crackers one at a time and eat one before you prepare the next.)

- Nachos made with 1 ounce of fat-free tortilla chips or a crisp baked pita, salsa, fat-free bean dip, and low-fat cheese

- 4 cups of air-popped popcorn

- An artichoke with low-fat dressing or salsa as dip

- A baked apple

54. Keep seconds a safe distance away.

See tool 170 in the Behavior Tools chapter.

Tools for High-Risk Times: You Don't Have to Blow It

CHOCOLATE CRAVINGS: GUILTLESS GRATIFICATION

55. Satisfy your chocolate urge—safely.

When only chocolate will do, indulge in the following lower-calorie, lower-fat treats.

- A snack-size candy bar

- A small peppermint patty

- A fudge pop

- A frozen peeled banana dipped in chocolate syrup

- Hot cocoa

- Chocolate sorbet with 1 tablespoon of chocolate syrup

56. Take a chocolate-appreciation break.

This tool, created by Dr. David Sobel, author of *The Healthy Mind, Healthy Body Handbook*, is about engaging all of your senses—sight, smell, touch, and so on—to fully appreciate the oral ecstasy that is chocolate. Give it a try—you might find that *one* piece of the finest chocolate is all you need when you follow these eight steps.

1. Appreciate the chocolate's beautiful dark color.

2. Feel the weight and smooth texture as you gently toss it in your hand.

3. Slowly inhale its rich aroma.

4. Take the smallest bite you can and extract as much taste as possible. The first bite coats the palate.

5. Take a larger bite. Feel how it melts from a solid to a liquid in your mouth.

6. Savor the creamy feel of the chocolate and the intense flavor as it melts at precisely body temperature.

7. Swallow and enjoy the lingering aftertaste.

8. To prolong the pleasure, slowly sip a cup of warm water. It fills you up and cleanses your palate so you won't want to eat more.

57. End premenstrual pig-outs, part 1.

Does your chocolate gene kick into high gear just before your period? Try this. Portion out 300 calories' worth of a starchy food, such as cereal, popcorn, or crackers, into little plastic bags, in one-serving portions. Eat one bagful every 90 minutes or so until dinner.

58. End premenstrual pig-outs, part 2.

If munching starches doesn't work, opt for a very, very spicy food, such as five-alarm salsa. Spicy fare has been known to short-circuit even the most serious chocolate jones. Go ahead, eat it with a spoon. If you can.

NIGHT EATING: SHUT DOWN THE P.M. MUNCHIES

59. Start with a salad.

When you get home from work, eat a large salad with low-fat or fat-free dressing. (Prepare the salad fixings ahead of time and don't forget to measure out the dressing.) Then have the rest of your dinner later. Don't scarf it down, either. Try to use some of the other tools you've come across. Drink seltzer with a wedge of fresh lemon from a wine glass; eat at the dining-room table.

60. Save your starch.

If you regularly eat a baked potato, rice, or other starch at dinner, save it. Then enjoy it when your night hungries kick in.

61. Split up your meal.

Eat half of your dinner when you get home and eat the other half at 9:00 P.M.

62. Delay your gratification.

Rather than nibble tasteless food because it's lower in calories, allow yourself to have one after-dinner snack that you really, really want, such as one sliver of cheesecake. Then delay eating it for as long as you can. The longer you wait, the closer you get to your bedtime, which is usually the signal to stop eating.

Again, use some of your other tools to help you. Enjoy your dessert without the benefit of your favorite TV sitcom and brush your teeth afterward, to signal that you're finished with food for the night.

63. Close the calorie "gate."

This is what I call a bridge tool—one that gets you through until you can automatically opt for more supportive behaviors.

Decide how many calories you want to consume in a certain time period—let's say, from 9:00 to 11:00 P.M. Then, in that period, eat your fill of the lowest-calorie foods possible.

Try bowls of cantaloupe, lettuce leaves, or raw sweet peppers. Eat as much as you wish throughout the night.

64. Ice your appetite.

You can also opt for sugar-free ices or Popsicles. Go ahead. Eat 10 if you must. This, too, is a bridge tool. So use it only until you can confine your eating to discrete meals and snacks.

65. Float away.

After dinner, immediately drink a liter of water. It can put the kibosh on those nightly urges to nibble.

66. Fatten up your dinner.

Food that contains fat is more satiating—that is, it makes you feel fuller longer. Fat also makes food taste better. (Duh.)

If you now subsist on low-fat or fat-free everything, add some fat to your meal, such as a slice of cheese or a 3-ounce broiled hamburger. You may feel satisfied longer—and you won't need to nibble on a snack later on.

67. Dine on a meal replacement.

The theory here: If you're going to eat later anyway, reduce the calories of your main meal.

Tools for Social Occasions:
Celebration without Temptation

BARHOPPING, BUFFETS, COCKTAIL PARTIES:
STAY-SLENDER STRATEGIES

68. Order first, drink later.

Place your order before you have your glass of wine. Alcohol loosens our inhibitions, which makes us less careful about overeating.

69. Nix the screwdrivers and Kahlúas.

Avoid drinks made with fruit juices or cream. Both pack a mother lode of calories.

70. Try a virgin Bloody Mary.

That's a Bloody Mary without the vodka. The spiciness of the tomato juice will fill you up, and you'll get to munch on celery, too.

71. Imbibe by half.

Alternate your drink of choice with a glass of club soda garnished with a wedge of lemon or lime. You may save hundreds and hundreds of calories.

72. Picture a piranha in the peanut bowl.

Sitting at the bar? Keep your hand out of the peanuts. They're 800 calories a cup—or 200 calories a grab. To keep your fingers out of the bowl, imagine that there's a piranha in it waiting to bite off your fingers.

73. Choose hors d'oeuvres or dinner.

If you attend a function that includes a cocktail/hors d'oeuvres hour followed by a sit-down dinner, decide *before you go* whether to eat just the hors d'oeuvres or the dinner.

If it's the hors d'oeuvres you want, pop mints during dinner or leave after the salad course. If you opt for the dinner, consider skipping the cocktail hour or arriving fashionably late.

If you want to attend both, map out your strategy before you go. For example, you might decide that you'll have one alcoholic drink and three hors d'oeuvres, followed by dinner. So pace yourself and decide which hors d'oeuvres you'll choose—perhaps only low-calorie foods such as sushi or raw veggies.

This is a good time to use some of your Behavior Tools. The first? Sit as far away from the food as you can.

RESTAURANT MEALS: DINING OUT WITHOUT FILLING OUT

74. Master the bread basket.

When it comes to restaurant dining, one of the thorniest problems to confront the weight-conscious is the Bread Basket Dilemma. We all know we shouldn't eat the bread—or at least, not the whole basket. The question is: How?

This tool allows you to decide how you'll handle this dilemma even before you get to the restaurant. Best of all, you have choices. (You can adapt this tool for use at Mexican and Chinese restaurants, which often proffer bowls of taco chips or deep-fried noodles).

- Ask your waitperson not to bring bread.

- If you'll be at a restaurant where you know the bread is especially good, ask your waitperson to serve everyone individually (in case one person wants more than one serving).

- Bring a pack of sugarless gum so you can work your jaws while you wait for your meal.

- Eat it only if it's whole grain.

- Eat the bread only with your meal.

- Have it as your main meal with a salad.

- Eat it only if it's warm.

- Ask that a plate of raw veggies be put in front of you at the same time the bread is served.

- Delay eating it for as long as you can. Once you start, it's harder to stop.

75. Order from the invisible menu.

Chances are you go to the same few restaurants over and over again, so you already know what's on the menu. So why open it and tempt yourself with the dishes you know you shouldn't eat? The trick: Pretend you don't see the menu. It's invisible. Now, order the low-fat, low-calorie healthy fare you know is inside. Things like a turkey sandwich on rye with lettuce, tomato, and mustard, with a cup of bean soup. Or the grilled salmon with baby red potatoes (hold the butter) and a tossed green salad (low-cal dressing on the side). When you use the invisible menu, the double nachos and the Reuben sandwiches are out of sight— and off your plate.

76. Say "steamed, please."

Get into the habit of ordering veggies that are steamed rather than drenched in butter or oozing with cheese sauce. It never hurts to be reminded that steamed veggies are nutritious, low in calories, and most important, filling. If you don't see them on the menu or on the blackboard that lists the specials, ask. While some restaurants drench their vegetables of the day in butter or cheese sauce, others will accommodate your request.

77. Make portions a no-brainer.

If you go to a restaurant that typically serves huge portions, ask your waitperson if you can have a half-size portion. If not, ask him or her to wrap half your entrée before even setting your plate in front of you. Save it for tomorrow's lunch.

78. Or share a sinful entrée.

Want that forbidden portion of fettuccine Alfredo? Ask a dinner companion if he would like to split it. Don't be embarrassed. Perhaps he wants to splurge, too, and will gladly take you up on your offer.

79. Hydrate while you wait.

While you wait for your meal to arrive, sip tall glasses of ice water rather than an alcoholic beverage. You'll not only get your daily requirement of H_2O but be more likely to exercise restraint. (Alcohol loosens our inhibitions, which makes it more likely for us to think, "The heck with it!" and order the death by chocolate cake for dessert.)

80. End your meal the European way.

If you're still hungry, enjoy fresh fruit for dessert. If you don't see it on the menu, ask for it anyway. Many restaurants use fresh oranges, grapes, cantaloupe, and strawberries as a garnish. And most chefs will gladly accommodate your request.

The Mood Tools

Everyday Tools: Expand Your Mind, Downsize Your Body

81. Write your way to better control.

"Self-monitoring"—the clinician's term for keeping a diary—is one of the most effective treatments for overweight and obesity. And while not everyone enjoys writing down what and how much she eats, how much activity she gets, or the emotions she feels, the fact remains: It works.

Keeping a diary helps you track your progress, record your triumphs, and set and meet goals, which can send your motivation soaring. It also allows you to identify your weaknesses, so you can change them. And *that* makes you feel like you're mastering your weight problem, instead of the other way around.

Hate tallying calories and fat grams? Don't. See The Ultimate Weight-Loss Weapon: A Pen on page 203 for more information on how to set up a food diary that's right for *you*.

82. Learn to discern hunger.

Are you really hungry, or do you just want to eat? Sometimes, it's hard to tell. Here's a hint: True hunger is accompanied by specific physical sensations, such as headache, light-headedness, or a gnawing feeling in your stomach.

If you're not sure whether your hunger is physical or psychological, don't eat until you experience one of the symptoms above. Ask yourself if you're physically in need of food.

Will you have to wait all day? I doubt it. Will it hurt you to try? No. (Unless you have a health condition that might put you at risk, such as diabetes. Then ask your physician if you can try this tool.) If you don't know when you're hungry, how will you know when you're full?

83. Tout your smallest triumphs.

View your progress as a series of small wins, rather than as one huge victory. This attitude adjustment will help you steer clear of all-or-nothing thinking, which is a mutant strain of perfectionism.

Count any and all improvements you've made in your eating or workout program as small wins. You're overeating less? Small Win #1. You didn't finish that piece of chocolate cake? Small Win #2. You walked a quarter of a mile longer than you thought you would? Small Win #3. And so on. Every day look for those tiny triumphs—and respect them.

84. Stop with the "shoulds" and "musts."

When it comes to weight control, they're some of the most damaging words in the English language. "Should" is judgmental, while "must" sets the stage for rebellion.

Do this. Each time you think, "I should have . . . ," stop. Then say, "Maybe next time I'll try to. . . ." And every time you think, "I must . . . ," tell yourself you *could*. Or *might try*. That way, the surly teen rebel in you gets to save face.

85. Always decide to eat.

More often than not, we don't consciously decide to eat. The food is there, and our mouths and jaws go on autopilot. But when you *decide* to eat, you make a conscious decision to feed yourself.

Use the following guidelines to help you eat with your full consent.

Sitting down means deciding to eat. Foods we eat standing up are usually those we feel we're not allowed to savor.

Dressing up your table means deciding to eat. The experience of a meal changes when you sit down to a table dressed with matching tablecloth and napkins and perhaps an inexpensive bouquet of flowers or candles as a centerpiece. Treat yourself with the same courtesy you would a guest in your home.

Eating without distractions means deciding to eat. When you eat in front of the TV or computer screen, while reading, or behind the wheel of your car, you haven't chosen to eat. You've let your activity dictate your eating behavior. A commercial break, turning the pages of a book, or getting into your car for a long trip or your daily commute can trigger the desire for food. But physical hunger is the best reason to eat. So keep eating entirely separate from other activities.

Eating slowly means deciding to eat. Put down your fork between bites. Chew thoroughly. As you eat, frequently ask yourself, "How does this taste?" and "Am I hungry?" Then actually answer. Above all, savor whatever you're eating.

86. Nurture the skin you're in.

If you use food as a reward for a job well done, start a new habit: Lavish small but satisfying gifts on your body. They don't have to be expensive. They just have to be special, like new nail polish in a vibrant color, a fragrant new aftershave or cologne, or a salon pedicure. Gifts like these can help you begin to treat your body with respect and to give it pleasure.

87. Dress in living color.

If you hide your body in dark, drab colors, here's one way to develop body confidence: Add a shot of color to your wardrobe. If it makes you feel uncomfortable to wear a lot of color, start small, perhaps with a silk scarf in an exquisite shade of magenta or orange. If you feel really brave, go out on a limb with a pair of funky blue-suede shoes. See if you want to work your way up to a jacket or pantsuit in your favorite hue.

If you find that you're reluctant to add color to your wardrobe, bring a friend with you when you shop to give you feedback and encouragement.

Staying the Course: Tools to Keep You Going Strong

88. Go for the goals.

You've probably read that it's important to set goals when you follow a weight-control program. Problem is, not many of us know how to do it right. Here's how to set goals that work.

■ The more specific your goals, the more likely you are to meet them. A vague goal (such as "I want to lose 20 pounds") or one that is too hard to reach precisely (such as "lose 20 pounds in 8 weeks") suddenly seems more doable when it's rewritten as "For the next month, I will try to eat close to 1,500 calories a day and walk from 6:00 to 6:30 P.M. on Mondays, Wednesdays, and Fridays."

■ Don't set goals that smack of all-or-nothing thinking. For example, it may not be helpful to set an absolute weight goal such as "I am going to lose 4 pounds this month." What happens if you lose 3 pounds but feel that you got a handle on your night eating?

■ Break goals into two categories: long-term goals, which may take 6 or more months to achieve, and short-term goals, which you can accomplish in weeks or a few months. Meeting your short-term goals gives you a sense of pride and accomplishment that will keep you moving toward your long-term goals.

■ Give each goal a deadline, then use that date to keep yourself on track.

■ Make sure your goals are achievable, given your current level of fitness, your age, and your body type. Setting impossible goals is no better than not setting any at all.

■ Don't label yourself a failure if you don't meet your goals. Making achievable goals is a *skill*, which means it must be learned. Realize that you always have another opportunity to make more realistic ones.

■ To refresh your motivation, revise your long-term goals quarterly and your short-term goals regularly.

89. Play the "what's in it for me?" game.

When you're staring temptation in the face, stare it down by asking yourself this question: "How will this [third slice of pizza, giant cinnamon bun, bacon cheeseburger] help me? And how might it hurt me?"

Don't just ponder the question. Actually write down your answers. (If you're out in public, you can always go to the ladies' room and do it. It won't take more than a minute or two.)

Your list might look something like this:

How it will help me

It will improve my mood. I'll like that feeling of intimacy and festivity.

It will give me something to enjoy. I'll get to savor the utter deliciousness of a fat-laden food.

I won't have to worry about going off my diet. I won't care what else I eat for the rest of the evening, and I'll have a better time.

It will take my mind off my worries.

How it will hurt me

It will affect my mood. If I give in, I'll feel guilty, ashamed, and depressed.

It will affect my motivation. If I give in to this [pizza, cinnamon bun, cheeseburger], I might say, "What the heck," and abandon my program. I've done it before.

It may cause me to gain weight.

It may affect my blood pressure, blood sugar, or blood cholesterol.

When you actually write it down, it's easier to see that the object of your desire is more likely to hurt you than help you, which may make it easier to say, "No thanks."

90. Use the "envelope, please!" tool.

Decide on your long-range goal. Write it out, put it in an envelope, seal the envelope, and tape it to your refrigerator door. Keep it there for the duration of the goal—6 months, 9 months, 1 year. Then rip open the envelope to assess how close you've come to meeting it.

91. Make a "goal map."

Creating a goal map can help you assess where you are in terms of meeting your goals, see the progress you've made, and plan what you should do next to meet your goals. It's a great tool because it helps you see what's working for you as well as what you need to work on. Plus, you get to play. Give yourself plenty of time . . . and permission to have fun!

Assemble scissors, old magazines, crayons, watercolors, pastels, Magic Markers, colored paper, paste, glitter . . . any material that helps you access your creative side.

Ask yourself the following questions: What weight would I like to reach and maintain? What do I need to learn to help me reach my goals? How will I motivate myself and monitor my eating behavior? What should I eat more or less of to improve my health? What kinds of physical activity might I like to pursue, and how do I start?

With those questions in mind, lay out a large sheet of blank paper. Using your materials, choose or draw an image to serve as the center, or "wheel," of your goal map. Then choose or draw images that serve as its "spokes"—the actions you now take or plan to take to meet your goals. Some spokes might include a tape measure that represents your ideal measurements, a vegetable garden to represent your new eating habits, and magazine photos of exercises or activities you plan to begin. Use as many spokes as you wish.

You might conceive of your goal map as a road map that leads to your final destination, with milestones and weight-maintenance techniques dotting the route. Or as a tree. The roots can represent your core weight-maintenance goals and principles, and the leaves can be the goals and tools that will get you there.

Jane, one of my clients, had lost 40 pounds and felt terrific. In fact, she'd just bought her first pair of bicycle shorts. To keep her motivation high as she continued to lose weight, she created a goal map. She used a photo of a model in bike shorts as her wheel. Her spokes were the tools she planned to use to stay in those shorts.

Jane cycled three times a week but wanted to work out 4 or 5 days a week. So she used one spoke for her cycling and another for the twice-a-week jog she planned to start. Her other spokes were a nutritious diet, a healthy body image, higher self-esteem, continuing to use her food diary, and reaching out for support.

92. Map your path to health.

This map, called the "road to health map," is similar to the goal map. It's just that you map your health goals rather than your weight goals. In this map, represent weight as only one of the many spokes or roads leading to good health. This is an especially helpful tool if you happen to have diabetes, high blood pressure, heart disease, high cholesterol, or another chronic disease that is affected by weight.

Chances are that after you do this tool, you'll feel pretty good about yourself. That's because when you make positive changes in your eating and activity level, your health often improves, even if your weight doesn't change.

93. Set a weight range.

Once you've achieved your goal weight, set a weight range. If you've lost 50 pounds or less, keep your range within 5 to 7 pounds. If you've lost 100 pounds or more, keep within 10 to 15 pounds.

94. Send out an SOS.

If you exceed your upper range but cutting calories and increasing your physical activity don't take off the weight, seek out support. Help might be in the form of Weight Watchers or TOPS (Take Off Pounds Sensibly) meetings or a dietitian or personal trainer you hire for a short period of time.

95. Challenge your beliefs about perfection.

To eat or not to eat? That is the question. And each of us attempts to answer it by forwarding it to our personal internal debating team.

Unfortunately, the team is sadly at odds. One member, the Kid, argues for our desires. Another, the Dictator, argues for control. We rarely hear from the Grown-Up, who argues for compromise.

At times, this internal debate becomes paralyzing.

The Kid: "I want it, and I'm gonna eat it!"

The Dictator: "If you eat it, you're bad. And to make up for your gluttony, I'll make you starve."

Often, the debate ends when we get tired of starving and eat everything in sight.

Had we listened for the Grown-Up, we might have heard, "I'm ending the debate right here. I'm fine with eating one or two servings of this, my favorite food. And that's the final word."

This tool will help integrate your internal debating team and allow the Grown-Up to say his or her piece.

Divide a piece of paper into three columns. Label the columns Dictator, Kid, and Grown-Up. Which team member is the loudest and most persistent today? What is each saying? Write down their dialogue.

Remember, the Grown-Up can compromise, making the Kid and the Dictator feel as if they each "won" the debate.

The Kid: "I want an entire chocolate cake to myself!"

The Dictator: "You're a glutton. I'm going to make you starve tomorrow."

The Grown-Up: "It's dangerous to bring a whole cake into the house. But if you want to go to the coffee shop or bakery around the corner and have a piece of cake with a cup of coffee, do it."

If it's difficult to use this tool, pretend you're talking to a friend who is "awfulizing" in front of you and that you must help her see the bigger picture.

96. Tally up your positive changes.

When you're on a weight-loss or weight-maintenance program, it's vital to focus on the positive changes you're making rather than on the weight you've lost. This tool gives you the chance to rate your small successes on your way to your long-term goals.

Read the list of items on the following pages. Each has a point allotment. (The points add up to 35.) Consider your progress for each item, then award yourself a point value based on the number in the point-allotment category. (Yes, you can award yourself half-points!)

When you're done, add up your points. The closer you are to 35, the better you're doing. Most likely, you'll find that you're never doing as badly as you think you are. Remember that this tool measures progress as success. So tally up. Maybe in one category, you progressed from 0 points to ½ point. Good for you!

Activity Level

If you're performing the activities below in accordance with your goal, give yourself the point. Award yourself a half-point if you're performing the activity but not as often as your goal.

Strength training (lifting weights) _____

Aerobic activity (walking, jogging) _____

Other activity (Pilates, yoga, tai chi) _____

Social activity (dancing, tennis) _____

Watching less TV _____

Increasing everyday activity _____

Quality of Life

Can you do things you never could before? Do you feel happier, more content, more confident? Give yourself a point.

I can walk for longer periods of time. _____

I can sit in a theater or bus seat. _____

I can bend more easily to pick up things. _____

I'm more comfortable with my eating at home. _____

I'm more comfortable with my eating in restaurants. _____

I'm generally feeling better about myself. _____

I sit less because it's easier to move. _____

My clothes fit better. _____

I feel more social. _____

Eating Patterns and Behaviors

How have your eating habits and behaviors changed for the better?

My eating pattern is stable during the week. ____

My eating pattern is stable on weekends. ____

I stay within my calorie goal on weekdays. ____

I stay within my calorie goal on weekends. ____

I make healthier food choices than I used to. ____

Differentiating between Physical and Psychological Hunger

Are you learning the difference between physical hunger and "mood hunger"?

I eat only when I'm physically hungry. ____

I don't eat when I am not hungry as often as I used to. ____

I don't usually eat to numb my feelings anymore. ____

I can leave food on my plate. ____

I don't eat food if it doesn't taste good. ____

My eyes are no longer bigger than my stomach. ____

Health Improvements

If you're in perfect health, award yourself the whole point.

My blood pressure has improved. ____

My blood glucose has improved. ____

My blood cholesterol has improved. ____

My LDL cholesterol has improved. ____

My serum triglycerides have improved. ____

I am taking less medication than I used to. ____

My EKG has improved. ____

My arthritis is improved. ____

Other ____

97. Visualize your hunger.

You don't need artistic talent to create a visual scale. For some people, a visual scale is a less judgmental way to record their food intake. But you can use it to quantify anything from your degree of fullness to your satisfaction before and after a meal or your feelings of guilt after eating.

To use it, simply draw a line that indicates where you fall on the scale. This is what a visual scale rating fullness looks like.

Not full——————————————————————— Full

One of my clients didn't pay attention to the fullness signals her body sent. Her signal for being full? When the food was gone.

I suggested that she might feel full sooner if she took heed of what being full felt like. I then asked her to use the visual scale to rate her degree of "fullness." She rated it before she began her meal and stopped eating when she could mark three-quarters of the line or more, even if food was still available. The scale helped her become more aware of what being "full" felt like, so she could stop eating before she felt stuffed.

98. Try the body beautiful exercise.

If you're a woman, chances are you've stood in front of a mirror more than once, berating your belly, butt, or thighs. This tool can help you come to view your body as a sophisticated machine, rather than a mass of flaws.

Change into loose, comfortable clothing and remove your shoes. Lie on your back on your bed, a mat, or the carpet.

Close your eyes. Wiggle your toes. One at a time, lift your feet slightly and move your feet in circles, then up and down. Then drop your foot back onto the surface and relax. Hone in on your toes and feet. How do they feel? Do you like their size and shape? Could you take better care of them? If so, how? Perhaps you might get regular pedicures, treat yourself to a weekly foot massage, splurge on a whirlpool-type foot bath. Maybe you could wear a toe ring or ankle bracelet.

Give your calves, thighs, hips, bottom, waist, abdomen, breasts, arms, back, neck, shoulders, and face the same kind of loving but detailed scrutiny. Instead of lifting, briefly tighten and then relax the muscles of each of these areas in turn. Be candid (yet not harsh) about the areas you don't like, but acknowledge the good.

Be realistic, too. Don't compare your body with that of a celebrity or even a friend or family member. Recognize that every part of your body works hard and deserves praise and pampering.

99. Don't sneak your eats.

If you are a closet eater, take a risk: Eat in full view of friends and family. This simple action conveys a powerful message: "I have chosen to eat." And even if you eat something you wish you hadn't, like a slice of your sister's homemade blueberry pie, you can feel proud that you made a choice rather than crumbling in the face of a craving. When you exercise your right to choose, you have power. And when it comes down to whether or not to eat, you always, always have a choice.

100. Build yourself up.

When you continually run yourself down, you tear your self-esteem to shreds. And tattered self-esteem can lessen your chances of losing weight or maintaining your weight loss. This tool can help you rethink the way you view yourself and boost your self-esteem.

Grab a sheet of paper and list at least five positive qualities that describe you. (By all means, list more than five!) Some possibilities:

> Smart
> Sensitive
> Creative
> Funny
> Compassionate
> Generous

Now, come up with your own.

Study your list. Note that most of these qualities aren't dependent on your weight.

Now, ponder this: While there are parts of the external you that you'd like to improve, the internal you is pretty good just as it is.

101. Practice mindfulness.

Techniques that connect the mind to the body, such as meditation, can be extremely helpful as you strive to shed extra pounds or maintain your goal weight. They relax your body as they calm your mind, allow you to disconnect from the stressors of daily life, and let your body rest and recharge.

Try this very simple meditation: Sit quietly in a comfortable position, preferably with your back straight. Focus your mind on your breath, on a silently repeated sound, or on a stationary object like a flower, paperweight, or candle flame. As you focus your mind, allow all other thoughts to float away, gently refocusing as many times as necessary.

Practice for 15 to 20 minutes every day if possible. Try to meditate just before the time period when you tend to overeat the most. Also, try to meditate at the same time every day, which can help reinforce the habit.

Tools for High-Risk Situations: Staying Calm and in Control

102. Face down body woes.

It's only natural to avoid situations that make you feel bad about your body, such as shopping for clothes or looking at yourself in the mirror. Sometimes, they can make us feel so bad that we console ourselves with food.

To help you face your body issues, pick one thing that you tend to avoid—perhaps wearing a bathing suit. Then take small steps to conquer that fear.

First, just buy the suit. The next day, wear it around the house for 10 minutes. Later, wear it in front of your partner. Eventually, you may feel comfortable enough to swim laps or join a water aerobics class.

103. Play the "I'd rather be . . ." game.

You know those bumper stickers that read "I'd rather be golfing" or "I'd rather be fishing"? They're popular, I think, because reading them gives you a momentary pause of pleasure. For a split second, you *are* on the links or in the stream. This tool tries to replicate that brief "pleasure zone."

So when the stress is closing in and it seems that only a jelly doughnut from the break room will restore your equilibrium, stop the panic thoughts and complete this sentence: "I'd rather be . . ."

Some examples:

> "I'd rather be sitting in the sun, on a blanket in the middle of a field."

> "I'd rather be curled up on my bed, taking a long, long nap."

> "I'd rather be sipping a steaming cup of coffee as I work the crossword puzzle in the Sunday *New York Times Magazine*."

Note how calm you are and that your appetite is under control. Practice this mental exercise each day.

104. See how skillful you are.

When you feel frustrated and discouraged, you need to realize that you *can* succeed. To help convince you—quickly—sit down and make a list of the skills you have that can help you make your weight-loss or maintenance program a success. List skills such as "I'm a hard worker," "I manage my time well," or "I'm a fast learner." Then brainstorm ways you can use these skills to meet your goals.

105. Don't lighten up until you're ready.

Some people shed extra pounds quite happily until they hit a certain weight. Then, they get scared. They may fear that losing more weight will release their sexuality. Or that by losing weight, they are less powerful. If this sounds like you, you're at a critical point in your weight-control program.

If you fear losing more weight—even if your current weight is quite high—set one goal: to maintain your weight instead of losing or regaining it. (Most people know how to lose and gain weight; few understand how to *maintain* it.) Remind yourself that you can always start losing again when you feel ready.

I had a patient who, despite being seriously obese and losing an initial 50 pounds, was afraid to break the 400-pound mark. I told her to stay at that weight until she felt ready to lose more. In the past, she would have regained the 50 pounds and then some. Now, she was free to *stop* losing weight and resume only when it felt "right." And as she waited for the right time, she could take pride in having the courage to keep those 50 pounds off.

106. Play the "how many calories could I eat?" game.

Some of us are Awfulizers, which means that we tend to turn a minor slip, such as one afternoon or one day of overeating, into a major catastrophe. At the same time, we minimize the ways we've stuck to our program, such as keeping to our workout schedule or ignoring the doughnuts in the coffee room at work.

If we're not careful, awfulizing can make us feel so terrible that we think, "The heck with it!" and abandon our program. The following tool can help us put slips into perspective so we don't let them undermine our progress.

Make a list of everything you would eat on your worst pig-out day. French fries, ice cream, pizza, a double order of nachos, moo shu pork, you name it.

Spend no more than 2 minutes contemplating the calorie count of this one-day blowout. It's rather enormous, right? Thousands of calories, right?

Now, consider this. Those thousands and thousands of calories might translate to 2, maybe 3 pounds on the scale. Who among us hasn't gained or lost that much?

The take-home message here is: One day of overeating isn't as bad as a week. One week of overeating isn't as bad as a month. You get the picture. Just stop overeating as quickly as you can. This may be a good time to tackle the very next tool.

107. Do a weekly review.

When you feel like you're losing your battle with food, try the simple self-assessment below. It can help you see how you're undermining your goals, as well as the positive, healthful steps you're taking. Feel free to use this tool daily if you need to.

Answer the questions "yes" or "no."

_____ I overate on high-fat, high-sugar foods but continued to eat healthy ones, too.

_____ I overate but stuck to healthier foods even when I overate.

_____ I tried a new tool when I realized I was overeating.

_____ I need to find a more effective tool or tools.

_____ I've reviewed the tool chapters and am testing a new tool.

_____ If I noticed I was thinking negatively about myself or my weight, I tried to think in a more positive way.

_____ I reached out for support.

_____ I feel better now that I've filled out this self-assessment.

Complete the following statement.

One small thing I can do to help myself is _____
_____.

108. Use the "tell it like it is" tool.

Sometimes, we want to explode—to yell, to scream, to let the world know about who or what has hurt or angered us. But too often, we stuff down those screams with food because we fear confronting our anger or the person who's angered us. This tool can help you let out what's eating you before you eat everything that isn't nailed down.

Every time you perceive that you're eating out of anger, write down why you're eating, what you're eating, and how and why it will satisfy you.

Here's an example: "I'm sick of being overworked, underpaid, and unappreciated. My boss off-loads project after project and expects me to stay late, while she leaves early. I hate her. I am eating this entire fat-free cake because I need my job and I don't feel strong enough to tell her how angry I feel. I am eating because I want to take off her head."

Now, ask yourself what would happen if you didn't eat. Write it down. Would you go crazy? Would your boss somehow know how you felt? Would you take off someone else's head—your partner's, perhaps?

This tool makes it more difficult to punish yourself with food. Further, it allows you to see that you *can* cope with anger in ways that don't involve eating. And no matter how angry you are, you can feel better about this: You didn't use food in a way that made you feel bad.

109. Before you dig in, write a dissertation.

You know that immediately after you eat that half-jar of peanut butter or the remains of the half-gallon of ice cream, you'll feel guilty and ashamed. But still, the food beckons. Before you answer its call, use this stalling technique.

Grab a piece of paper (perhaps in a notebook reserved just for this purpose) and write out what you think eating this food will do for you. What are the benefits? What do you gain?

Some possible answers: It will alleviate my physical hunger. It will provide a temporary respite from my chronically stressful life. It will substitute for telling off my partner or snapping at my kid. It will give me something to do.

But don't stop at just one sentence. Try to write at least a paragraph and see what you find under that desire to eat. Sadness? Anger? Boredom? See if, as you write, the urge to eat passes.

110. Make a 911 call.

Before you dive into that cherry-cheese strudel you bought for company, call a friend and tell her what you're about to do. This "confession" accomplishes two important things. First, it legitimizes the eating because you admitted to the desire, loud and proud. Second, the act of telling often weakens the "need" to eat.

111. Play the sleep-cure game.

Imagine there was a magic spell that could put you to sleep during the 2 or 3 most difficult hours of your food day. When would that time be?

(Even if you feel that the whole day is out of control, you can probably pick one period of time that is the most difficult.)

Once you identify your high-risk time, schedule any nonfood activity to fill that period. Some ideas:

- Meet friends at a bookstore.

- Take a bike ride in the park.

- Go to the gym.

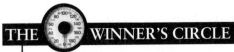

"INCORPORATING ACTIVITY IN MY DAILY LIFE HAS BEEN KEY"

Natalie Novod uses two key tools to maintain a 50-pound weight loss and get her around the Big Apple. Tool No. 1? Her right foot. Tool No. 2? Her left.

"Incorporating activity in my daily life has been key," says Novod, 51, a special education teacher. "I walk most every place unless I'm in a huge rush or there's very bad weather. I wouldn't consider *not* walking."

Novod walks a mile to and from the kindergarten-through-8th-grade school where she teaches and walks to do her shopping. In her quest to lose another 20 to 30 pounds, she's so focused on movement that she's memorized that 30 blocks is equal to about 1½ miles.

Novod's other key tools are designed to battle the night munchies. To keep her hands busy, she took up knitting again. Another favorite hobby that keeps her fingers flying is making beaded jewelry. "There's always another row to knit, another piece of jewelry to do, and that keeps me distracted (from eating)," Novod says.

A nearly empty refrigerator also serves to keep nighttime eating at bay. "I don't have a lot of food in the house," Novod says. "I keep on hand only those things that can't do me major harm, like yogurt or those salad mixes." Bottled water stashed in the refrigerator also fills Novod up when she peers in the fridge looking for something to eat.

- Call someone.

- Take a long, hot bath or shower.

- Take a nap or turn in early.

If your most difficult time occurs at work:

- Try to schedule meetings during your difficult period.

- Call a friend at that time.

Once a committed nibbler who ate most of her calories from 3:00 P.M. right up to bedtime, Novod now sticks to three planned meals and single-portion snacks. Although Novod still thinks of a meal as "something social," she insists on sitting down to eat dinner even when she's all alone.

Self-talk at mealtime or any time cravings strike is also a key tool in Novod's weight-loss arsenal. Her new policy to just say, "No, I won't," to herself reflects a perseverance that was missing in myriad other attempts at weight loss. "It's a coming-of-age thing, I believe," Novod said. "It was just time (to lose weight). Enough."

The health dividends are more than just a lower number on the scale. Thanks to the weight loss, Novod takes a lower dose of blood pressure medication. Her cholesterol levels are down, and so are her blood sugar levels, which were once so high that Novod was considered a borderline diabetic. "The risk of heart attack and stroke from being overweight didn't shake me up, but the thought of losing my eyesight did," Novod says of blindness, a complication of diabetes. "I couldn't be blind."

"I have had no one among my friends and relatives give me a hard time. They have not undermined my efforts, either overtly or in unconscious ways," she adds. "They have been very supportive."

- Keep a pencil in your mouth while you work.

- If it's late afternoon, try tool 7: Make breakfast a "mini" or tool 50: Stretch your lunch.

- Eat a small, nutritious snack at lunchtime and have lunch in the late afternoon.

- Go for a quick stroll around the office or building.

- Bring celery and carrot sticks from home to munch on.

112. Put your appetite on disconnect.

When you feel your eating is out of control, that feeling can spiral until you feel powerless to stop it. The key is to disconnect—temporarily—from the activity of eating, so you can make a decision about whether you want to continue. Separating yourself from the table can buy you enough time to get a grip.

Some disconnecting techniques:

- Brush your teeth when you've finished what's on your plate.

- Get up from the table for a few minutes before serving yourself a second helping.

- When you start eating, set an alarm clock or egg timer for 5 minutes. When it buzzes, decide whether you're still hungry—and whether you want to continue to eat.

- Sip some water between bites.

- Have a family member take care of the leftovers or else walk around your home before returning to the kitchen to clean up.

- Clean your house. Sometimes, it will make you feel better and reduce your desire to eat.

The Move Tools

Everyday Tools: Fun (and Funny) Little Ways to Shake a Leg

113. Be a dancing fool.

Don't feel motivated to move? Put on your favorite tunes and bop around while you prepare dinner or wash dishes. Dancing can brighten your mood as it burns calories. In fact, you may get so revved up that you feel like working out after all.

114. Take three.

Choose to do at least three active things each week—and then do them. You might vacuum the carpets strenuously (or beat dusty rugs outside with a broom), wash all the windows on the first floor of your home, walk a lap around the entire mall when you go shopping, wash the car, or do some strenuous gardening (pull weeds, haul clippings, and so on).

115. Take a few flights.

How many steps do you climb each day? Every trip helps burn calories and strengthen leg muscles. In fact, just 5 minutes of climbing stairs burns 45 calories. Keep track of each flight you climb. You may opt to take the stairs instead of the elevator more often.

116. Channel surf with power.

With a strong piece of thin cord, attach a 2- or 5-pound dumbbell to your TV remote control. Every time you change the station, do a few reps.

117. Tune in, tone up.

If you exercise while you watch TV, do some interval training. That is, pick up the pace during each commercial break. Or pick a character on your favorite soap opera or sitcom and speed up for each 2- or 3-minute segment that he or she is on-screen.

118. Step lively.

Get a pedometer to measure how many steps you take each day. Every week, try to walk farther. Compete against yourself: If you walk 7,000 steps the first week, try for 7,500 the next. Tracking your progress can be super-motivating.

119. Time your workout right—at night.

Consider working out before dinner, if you can. There's some evidence that overweight folks don't feel hungry after a period of physical activity.

120. Work your way out of the kitchen.

If it keeps you out of the refrigerator, exercise *after* you eat dinner. (Remember, no tool is absolute, so choose the tool that works for *you!*)

121. Try nickel-and-diming it.

A lot of little activity can add up to a significant calorie burn. Try some of these surprisingly simple ways to get yourself moving.

At home:

- Hide your TV remote. Get up and change the channel. (Remember when we *had* to?)
- Use hand can openers instead of electric ones.
- Wash the dishes by hand rather than use the dishwasher.
- When you watch TV, get off the couch and walk up and down your stairs during every commercial break.
- Use your exercise bike or treadmill while you watch TV.
- Put items on higher shelves so you have to reach.
- Wherever you go, park at the farthest end of the lot.

At the office:

- Move the printer away from your desk so you have to get up to retrieve your pages.

- Move the fax away from your desk. Same reason.

- Change your chair to a nonrolling one.

- Every hour, take a 5-minute stroll around the hall.

Staying the Course:
Tools to Keep You Going Strong

122. Start sl-o-o-ow.

Don't do too much, too quickly. It's one of the fastest ways to end up back on the couch—or worse. You can begin with as little as 5 to 10 minutes of exercise 3 to 5 days a week. (Consult your doctor before you embark on any fitness program.)

Choose a comfortable pace so sore muscles won't discourage you from continuing. After a week or so, gradually increase either the length of time you exercise or the number of days a week. Slowly work up to 30 minutes most days of the week.

123. Exercise like a kid again.

What kinds of physical activity did you like to do as a kid? Use this tool to help you find new activities for your old playful self.

If you liked . . .

- Climbing trees: Try indoor or outdoor rock climbing.

- Yard games: Golf without the cart. A beginner? Go to a chip-and-putt course first. The holes are short, and most folks are beginners. Or try bowling, another hand-eye coordination game.

- Dodgeball: Volleyball. You're less likely to get hit, but it still takes hand-eye coordination.

- Gymnastics or cheerleading: The new-style aerobics classes, such as Latin, urban, and salsa-flavored routines.

■ Jump rope or hopscotch: Rebounding—that's aerobics on a trampoline. It provides a fun, nonimpact, jump-around workout.

124. Be a duffer.

Learn to golf or just hit the links more often. In one study, when 55 sedentary, middle-aged men golfed two to three times a week over a 5-month period, they burned an average of 1,750 calories per game, walked an average of 5 miles, lost 5 pounds, and increased their "good" HDL cholesterol by 5 percent. Plus, it's fun!

125. Find some sweat buddies.

If you're social by nature, pair up with a friend or a group of friends and work out together. When you say you'll meet a friend on the walking path or at the gym, you're less likely to skip your workout.

Make sure your buddy is really committed to the workout, can motivate you to get out the door when you don't want to, and can walk at the same pace or slightly faster than you. If you can't find a friend to work out with, look for fitness-minded folks in dance classes (swing, salsa, square dancing), on the golf or tennis course, in a martial arts class, or on the local softball team.

126. Get moving in every season.

Spring and fall are ideal for walking. But what to do when the thermometer dips below freezing? You can ski. You can ice-skate. (Or take skiing or ice-skating lessons.) You can rent a pair of cross-country skis or snowshoes, or you can go snow tubing. In the summer, join the Y and swim laps or take a water-aerobics class.

127. Walk in the rain—really.

Don't let a drizzle keep you from your daily walk. To weather the weather, dress in clothing that breathes. (Don't wear a plastic rain slicker; it will keep the rain out but trap sweat in.) Walk on asphalt or concrete and avoid slippery surfaces such as wet grass or mud. Use a hat or visor to keep the rain off your face and wear bright colors so motorists can see you.

128. Jump to it.

Jumping rope tones your hips, thighs, and butt; it's inexpensive; and you can do it virtually anywhere. Plus, its high intensity can help blast you off a plateau. (You can burn up to 200 calories in 15 minutes!) A good rope costs about $15. Get the beaded kind, which won't tangle. If you're a beginner, avoid weighted ropes. Wear aerobic or cross-training sneakers with good cushioning and jump on wood, grass, carpeting, or a mat. Avoid concrete, tile floors, and thick carpeting.

129. Put some fun in your burn.

If you're looking for a good time, so to speak, these 10 activities burn a mother lode of calories in an hour. Calorie burns are based on a 150-pound person.

- Jumping rope: 544
- Roller-skating: 476
- Bicycling: 408
- Swimming: 408
- Playing hopscotch with the kids: 340
- Ballroom dancing: 296
- Coaching your kid's soccer team: 272
- Paddling a canoe: 238
- Walking in the woods: 238
- Playing Frisbee: 204

130. Put up some resistance.

If you don't now do some form of resistance training, consider adding it to your exercise program. If you'd rather not join a gym, you can purchase inexpensive handheld dumbbells, ankle weights, or exercise bands. Before you go for it, make sure you know what you're doing. Team a pair of inexpensive handheld weights with a variety of toning videos or find a user-friendly gym and ask for pointers from the staff.

131. Make workouts a family affair.

Families rarely exercise together. Make your family the exception. There's so much you can do as a unit. You can hike, bike, walk, jog, or engage in a family swim at the local Y. If you have a large, extended family, you might also organize a softball or volleyball game.

Tools for High-Risk Situations: Lose the Excuses, Find the Commitment

132. Establish an "inspiration point."

Turn a small area in your kitchen, bedroom, or study into your personal shrine to fitness. If you're often in the kitchen, you might hang a cork bulletin board and cover it with inspiring articles clipped from fitness magazines, news articles about ordinary women who've achieved extraordinary fitness goals, and motivational quotes. If you have a home gym in your basement, cover one entire wall with photos of women in motion—walking, dancing, lifting weights.

133. Determine your prime workout time.

If you're ready to give up your workouts, consider whether it's the *time* that you work out that you hate. If you're a morning person, do you try to get in your run or a swim as the sun goes down? Or if you're a zombie before noon, do you work out at the crack of dawn? Work out when you're most likely to do it, even if you have to rearrange your routine a bit. Chances are you'll enjoy your exercise time a bit more.

134. Dress for exercise success.

Get dressed for your workout no matter how tired you feel or how sick to death you are of this whole exercise thing. Once you've slipped into your sweats and tied your sneaker laces, you may actually want to work out.

135. Schedule exercise appointments.

Schedule your workouts into your day. You can use your handwritten to-do list, a daily planner, or the scheduling software on your computer at work, just as you would schedule a hair appointment or a meeting. Also, schedule your other obligations around your workout, rather than the other way around.

136. Take the angst out of exercise.

If you're self-conscious about your body, exercise can be intimidating. To feel and look your best while you work out, invest in a few attractive pieces of workout wear. If you're size 14 or larger, look for the Junonia line, which makes supportive, stylish activewear in these sizes for aerobics, swimming, and more. Check out their Web site www.junonia.com.

137. Keep your eyes on the prize.

The benefits of exercise go far beyond looking good in a bathing suit. To drive home that point, set one or two health goals. Yours might be to lower your blood pressure or blood cholesterol or to reduce your blood-sugar level. Thus, you measure your progress with something besides clothing size. As a bonus, you'll appreciate your body on a whole other level.

138. Take a "where's Waldo?" walk.

If your daily walk is getting a bit lame, make it a game. Walk for as long as it takes for you to spot three red cars, then do some stretches. Look for all the letters of the alphabet—in order—on people's mailboxes and on street signs. Or pick up your pace until you reach the next stop sign, then slow down until you see another one.

139. Hire a personal trainer.

Your motivation is ebbing? To fire yourself up, hire a personal trainer. (It can be less expensive than you think.) Just make sure he or she is certified by the American Council on Exercise (ACE). To find one in your area, call (800) 825-3636 or log on to www.acefitness.org.

140. Shake up your routine.

Change where or when you exercise. It's a great way to give your workout a makeover, even if you stick to the same activity.

If you're bored to tears by your treadmill workout, step outside and find a wooded walking path. If your after-work routine has become too routine, turn in early and see what it's like to walk as the sun rises.

141. Motivate with money.

Put a dollar in a jar each time you work out. Ask your partner to match your donation. On the first of each month, spend your earnings on a

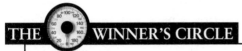

THE WINNER'S CIRCLE

"NOW I UNWIND WITHOUT EATING"

When Ruben Vazquez needs motivation to maintain a weight loss of more than 100 pounds, he simply opens his closet door and peeks inside.

"I look at all the new, thin clothes I bought," says Vazquez, a 38-year-old maintenance worker who once weighed nearly 400 pounds and dropped from a 54- to 40-inch waist. "Sometimes I even leave my new clothes out where I can see them," Vazquez says. "I look at them and tell myself, 'I fit into that, and I'm going to stay there.'"

Vazquez, a diabetic, also believes in the power of food diaries as much as the power of positive thinking. "If I eat at 8:00 P.M. and then I'm searching for something else again at 9:00, I look back at my diary and say, 'Hey, that's not real hunger. Something else must be going on,'" he says.

Exercise is another key tool in Vazquez's weight-loss arsenal. Six days a week he works out at a gym, combining biking, treadmill workouts, and other types of aerobic exercise with weight training and stretching. Nothing keeps him away.

"I do it because it's important to me," Vazquez says. "Sure, sometimes I don't feel like going, but I push myself to work out, and you know what? Afterwards, I feel so good, I could work another 8-hour shift all over again."

massage, manicure, or some new workout clothes. Alternately, if you do better with reinforcement, set aside $30 a month and *deduct* a buck every time you miss a workout.

142. Support a cause.

When your motivation to work is flagging, consider shaking a leg for someone other than yourself. Someone who could use your help. Support causes such as breast cancer, AIDS, or multiple sclerosis by entering fund-raising walks, bike rides, or runs. Beyond the exercise, you'll feel good about what you're doing. And you certainly won't be tempted to skip *this* particular "workout."

To quell cravings, Vazquez plans small portions of Fig Newtons and oatmeal raisin cookies, two of his favorite treats. At parties and holiday celebrations, he keeps a glass of carbonated water in his hands so he can't reach for calorie-laden goodies. If he simply must have something sweet, he reaches into his pocket for a peppermint candy. He uses the same techniques after a long day at work. "I can still unwind," Vazquez says, "but I unwind without eating."

When he slips up occasionally, Vazquez reminds himself that he is human and will get back on track again soon. "What I like about Cathy's approach is that she tells you to expect mistakes and that it's okay to fail sometimes," Vazquez says.

His hard work and determination have paid off. Thanks to the weight loss, his blood glucose levels have dropped so much that he no longer needs diabetes medicine.

Vazquez is determined to avoid the fate of his late father, a diabetic who lost both legs to the disease.

"I don't want to put my wife and son through what I went through," Vazquez says. "I don't think of this as being on a diet. This is a way of life for me. This *is* my life."

---

143. Make lifting more uplifting.

Can't wait to drop those dumbbells and get your weight training over with? These tips can help you find the fun in lifting.

- If you like camaraderie, join a strength-training class at a gym.

- If you prefer to go solo, lift in front of a mirror and focus on your form.

- Still bored? Haul your weights to the living room and work out while your stereo blasts your favorite music—Beethoven or rock and roll, it will rev you up.

144. Gear up.

Treat yourself to an inexpensive fitness gadget, such as a heart-rate monitor or pedometer. Tracking your workouts with devices like these can breathe new life into your same-old, same-old workout.

145. Get back in the saddle.

Many of us let one missed workout—or several—derail our fitness routines. Yet even the most dedicated exercisers occasionally get bored with their routines and go AWOL from the gym or their at-home fitness programs.

Don't feel overly guilty about workout "slips." Do whatever it takes to get back to working out. If you can, hire a personal trainer to jumpstart your program—and your motivation. If you can't afford to do that, call a fellow sweat buddy and ask if you can work out with her or him until you get back into the habit.

If you haven't worked out for more than 2 weeks, cut your routine in half and gradually work your way back. A shorter workout will ease you back into your routine. And you'll avoid sore muscles.

The Behavior Tools

Everyday Tools:
Use Your Head to Slim Your Bod

EATING AT HOME: MAKE EVERY MEAL A FEAST

146. Revisit your dining room.

We eat in bed, in the living room in front of the TV, in the study while we surf the Net. Yet we hardly ever partake in the one room designed exclusively for eating: the dining room, which is usually reserved for large family dinners or entertaining guests.

But imagine how much less we'd eat—and how much less frequently—if we confined our meals and snacks to this little-used room. We might think twice about having chips at 8:00 P.M. if we couldn't eat them in front of our favorite sitcom or nestled beneath our quilt with the latest John Grisham novel. We might also decide that if we're not willing to get up and eat our favorite snack at the dining-room table, there's probably no reason to eat it at all.

So make it a rule: Whether you're having breakfast or a 3:00 A.M. snack, eat at the dining-room table. Don't have a dining room? Eat only at the kitchen table.

147. Kick the talking heads out of your kitchen.

If you have a TV set in your kitchen, remove it. It's a primary cause of "eating amnesia"—forgetting that you ate, let alone how much.

When you switch off the TV, you accomplish two goals critical to weight control. One, you become aware that you're eating. Two, you become conscious of *how much* you're eating.

148. Make eating an event.

If you opt to eat all your meals at the dining-room table, gild the lily. Use your good china and cloth napkins. Buy fresh flowers for the table each week. Splurge on a set of beautiful candleholders. And eat everything—from a frozen diet entrée to a lone Oreo—slowly and with pleasure.

Why should you go to all this trouble? Because it turns a meal—or even a snack— into an event. And when you make each eating occasion an event, you become more conscious of how, what, and how much you eat. Consider this: Would you scarf an entire bag of chips if you had to put them on your best china, light your candles, and place your cloth napkin in your lap?

149. Have a seat.

There's a definite connection between being vertical and eating mindlessly. (Who among us hasn't eaten cold spaghetti from the pot over the kitchen sink or stood in the pantry crunching chips from the bag?) So unless you happen to enter a walkathon or dance marathon, you should never, ever eat standing up.

If you want that cold spaghetti, take it out of the pot, put it on a plate, and eat it at the dining-room table. If you want pretzels, put one serving in a small bowl and sit down at the dining-room table—not in front of the TV or in bed—to enjoy them. Sitting to eat will help you stay aware of how much you eat. Perhaps even more important, you'll be aware that you're eating in the first place.

EATING SLOWLY: THE NATURAL APPETITE SUPPRESSANT

150. Extend yourself.

Move your chair 6 inches or so from the table—enough so that you have to reach a bit to get at your plate. While you can't use this tool when you're in the midst of your meal, you *can* use it before the meal even starts. Simply lean back in your chair and cross your legs while others sip their drinks and munch bread and butter. What are you doing? You're relaxing. You also can use this tool to stay away from the leftovers so you won't be able to pick at them.

151. Turn meals into Monty Python skits.

Pick up a pair of chopsticks at a local Chinese place and use them at every mealtime for a week. Your all-thumbs awkwardness will force you to eat more slowly—and help you keep that message in mind. (You can also use a shrimp fork, if you like—same principle.) Once you've gotten the hang of eating more slowly, periodically break out the chopsticks to reinforce the message.

152. Divvy up your plate.

This tip comes from George Blackburn, M.D., a nutrition expert at Harvard Medical School: Visualize your dinner plate when it's filled with a moderate amount of food. Mentally divide the plate into four quarters. Take 10 minutes to eat the first quarter of your meal, even if it means you have to get up and walk around for a bit. Take 5 minutes to eat the next quarter. Take another 5 minutes to eat the third quarter. By that time, your brain should register that your stomach is full, and you might be able to skip the last quarter.

153. Eat in two acts.

Divide the food on your plate in half. (If you're dining out, make an imaginary dividing line.) Eat the first half of your meal. Stop eating and sip at a tall glass of water until it's empty. Are you still hungry?

If you want more food, eat the second half of your meal. If you're not sure, divide your remaining food in half. Eat half and drink another glass of water. Then decide whether you want the rest.

Another way to eat in two acts is to leave the table. If you're at home, eat half of your meal, then leave the table for 10 minutes. In that time, decide whether you're still hungry. In a restaurant, you can visit the restroom for 10 minutes or pretend you need to use the telephone.

154. Dilute your appetite 1.

Drink two glasses of water before a meal. The space the water takes up may reduce your hunger—and your food intake.

155. Dilute your appetite 2.

Eating a small amount of a high-fiber or high-protein food an hour before a main meal has helped some people reduce the amount they eat at that meal. Try an ounce of high-fiber cereal with fat-free milk or half of a small can of tuna.

MINDLESS EATING: PUT YOUR MIND WHERE YOUR MOUTH IS

156. Practice mindful mastication.

Do you take the time to chew your food thoroughly, or do you tend to swallow it too fast and almost whole? Really think about it. If you're a gulper, consciously try to chew more slowly. It can help you focus on what you're eating so you have the opportunity to enjoy it—or, if you're not enjoying it, to stop eating it.

157. Develop good taste.

Whether you're eating a double-pepperoni pizza or a crisp, crunchy apple, begin to become more aware of how food tastes. Ask yourself: How does this taste? Is this taste what I wanted? If it doesn't taste great, should I slow down my eating—or stop eating completely?

158. Brush away the picking.

When you're picking at a bit of this and a bite of that, hit the bathroom and brush your teeth. This tool gets you out of the kitchen and gives you something to do other than eat. Plus, that fresh, clean feeling may help blunt your urge to nibble.

159. Redefine "snack."

Most of us view a snack as an indulgence that falls outside the boundaries of good nutrition. It's time to change that view. A snack is:

- Smaller than a meal

- Eaten between meals

- A way to help balance your nutritional needs for the day

- Built into your daily food plan

- Eaten to appease hunger rather than boredom

Each time you reach for a snack, ask yourself if your choice meets one or more of these criteria. Chances are you may opt for an ounce of cheese and an apple or a can of water-packed tuna rather than a Big Grab bag of chips or a Snickers bar.

160. Use the tape trick.

Stick a wide strip of masking tape across the entrance to your kitchen at about waist or chest level between meals (or after dinner, if you're a night eater). It's an extremely effective way to make you conscious of how many times you find yourself heading into the kitchen for food.

161. Spray away work temptation.

Your colleague keeps a candy jar on her desk? The break room at work is constantly laden with homemade goodies? Stock up on breath spray and get into the habit of spritzing your mouth each time you leave your office or cube. You'll eventually associate using the spray with *not* eating those treats.

162. Reach for control.

Wind a string or a colorful bandage around one finger of your "eating hand" so you can see yourself reach for food. If you can *see* what you're doing, it can help you not to follow through on your impulse to eat.

163. Give mindless munching the white-glove treatment.

Instead of using string, pull on a glove. (Unless you're Michael Jackson, you might want to reserve this tool for at-home use only.)

164. Put your family on plate patrol.

If you scarf the scraps from your family's plates as you clear the table, teach your family to scrape their plates directly into the garbage can and take them to the sink or dishwasher. Then you can go on with your KP duties, temptation removed.

165. Or if you can't beat 'em, join 'em.

If you absolutely cannot resist finishing the remains of your children's mac and cheese, chicken fingers, or fish sticks, either at home or at a restaurant, have a salad with low-fat or fat-free dressing for dinner. Then have the rest of *their* dinner as your main course.

166. Try the papier-mâché tactic.

If you've ever made a papier-mâché puppet, you know how messy the wheat-paste-and-water concoction can be—and how busy it keeps your hands. And when your hands are occupied, they can't put food into your mouth. I rest my case.

Of course, you don't have to do papier-mâché. The goal is to keep your hands full of other things besides nachos and dip. Messy crafts or jobs work best. (Think sculpting clay, finger painting, digging in the garden, scrubbing the grout in the bathtub with a toothbrush.) If you get really desperate, give yourself a manicure. You can't eat half a bag of Oreos with wet nails.

PORTION CONTROL: CUT CALORIES—WITHOUT COUNTING THEM

167. Fool your eyes—and your appetite.

Replace your full-sized dinner plate with a sandwich plate. A smaller plate makes one serving look more substantial.

168. Attack portion drift.

Many of us who get close to our goal weights unconsciously start eating larger and larger portions. To get back on track, arm yourself with a measuring cup and a food scale and measure out portions every day for a week. Once you've reacquainted yourself with what one serving of rice or cereal actually looks like, measure or weigh your food choices one day a week to keep yourself honest.

169. Learn to eyeball portions.

See tool 36 in the Food Tools chapter.

170. Keep seconds a safe distance away.

When you put food right on the table, it's all too easy to reach for a second serving of mashed potatoes or another dinner roll. Worse, you may do it unconsciously. So keep platters, pans, and pots of food off the dining-room table and serve from the kitchen instead. To get a second helping, you must *choose* to go into the kitchen to get it—a choice you might not make if the food isn't right there in front of you.

171. Never eat from the source.

Food that's packaged in a large bag, can, box, or container is treacherous: There's no way to measure how much of it you're eating, and you're likely to eat far more than one serving.

To know *exactly* how much you're eating and to become more conscious of portion sizes, measure out one serving of the chips, beer nuts, ice cream, cheesecake, or whatever and put it in a dish or on a plate.

172. Play "keep away."

If your family habitually snacks on junk, don't just leave these foods in the cupboard and pantry to tempt you. Actively brainstorm ways to keep yourself away—far away—from others' goodies.

Be as creative as you can. Could you:

■ Stash the goodies in a basement nook or cabinet so they're not as readily accessible?

■ Ask your family to buy these foods as they crave them rather than have them in the house at all times?

■ Buy snacks for your family that you don't like?

173. Revisit your childhood.

Remember that GI Joe or Josie and the Pussycats lunchbox you loved so much? Well, *this* "lunchbox" can help you control your eating, day or night. If you tend to overeat during the day, pack your lunchbox with the food you want to eat between breakfast and dinner. (Now that you're out of grade school, feel free to opt for a small cooler or insulated lunch bag.)

You can eat it all in one sitting or space it out through the day. But when your lunchbox is empty, that's your signal to stop eating until dinner. If nighttime eating is your problem, assemble a nighttime lunchbox that includes your dinner plus your evening snacks. Just make sure your lunchbox fare doesn't exceed your allotted calories for the day.

Tools for Social Occasions: Mingle More, Munch Less

BARHOPPING, PARTIES, AND BUFFETS: PARTY ON WITHOUT FILLING OUT

174. Do the Cinderella thing.

If you plan to attend a cocktail party or a buffet-style dinner, arrive late, leave early—or both. If you arrive late, most of the good stuff will be gone by the time you show up. Leave early and you'll make it easier to avoid a second (or third) helping of dessert.

175. Stack the deck.

Next time you're invited to a party, offer to bring a vegetable tray and a low-fat dip. Your host will think you're a doll. And, of course, you are. But you also guarantee that there will be something at the party you can eat with abandon.

176. Keep your distance.

For obvious reasons, never stand or sit close to a buffet table. Park yourself at a table that's farthest away from those steam trays, where you can't see or smell the offerings.

177. Chew the right thing.

Whether you're at a party, buffet, or other social occasion, chew gum for as long as you can. (Just chew discreetly—no bubble blowing or obvious chomping.) You'll have to remove the gum to eat. Which is hard to do politely.

178. Master sleight of hand.

If you normally hold a fork in your right hand, hold your drink in your right hand and try to eat with your left (or vice versa if you're left-handed). You'll eat less—or at least make overeating more of a chore.

179. Follow the two-spoon rule.

At a buffet, don't put more than two different foods on your plate at a time. You can return to the buffet as often as you wish, but each time you finish what's on your plate, you'll have to make three decisions:

1. Whether you want more of the same food

2. Whether you want to try a different offering

3. Whether you want to go back at all

180. Or follow the one-plate rule.

Unlike the two-spoon rule, this tool allows you to put as many foods on your plate as you can fit. But you can't go back for seconds. (Of course, do exhibit some decorum. That one plateful shouldn't look like a mini Mount Everest.)

181. Choose hors d'oeuvres or dinner.

See tool 73 in the Food Tools chapter.

182. Find a restaurant role model.

If possible, try to sit next to the person who eats the least or who eats the slowest. He or she may help you to slow your own eating pace.

183. Order from the invisible menu.

See tool 75 in the Food Tools chapter.

184. Lead off the order.

Whether you're breaking bread with a lone companion or a whole group, be the first to order. It's easier to order a turkey sandwich—hold the fries—or the grilled fish and steamed asparagus when you don't have to listen to others opting for fettuccine Alfredo or the grilled Reuben and fries.

185. Order by proxy.

Feeling shaky? Have someone else in your party order for you. This is especially helpful if this person knows about and supports your weight-loss or weight-maintenance goals. Tell her what you want, then head to the restroom until you're sure the entire order has been placed.

186. Eat what you love, pare down the rest.

Before you enter a restaurant, decide what you really, really want. Then have it. Just reduce your intake of other foods you can live without.

Let's say you want the pasta carbonara. Ask your waitperson if you can order a half-portion. If not, request the half-portion anyway and pay for the whole. Then opt for salad with fat-free dressing on the side (or use a splash of balsamic vinegar) and a glass of seltzer instead of wine. Completely ignore the bread basket.

What *not* to do is opt for pasta with plain tomato sauce because it's lower in calories (when you really want the carbonara) but then add calories with bread, wine, salad dressing, and dessert.

187. Play the lifeboat game.

In the classic Alfred Hitchcock film *Lifeboat*, the survivors of a ship wrecked at sea must periodically toss a survivor overboard to keep the lifeboat afloat. This tool works along the same principle.

At a restaurant, choose *one* of the following three: alcohol, bread, or dessert. Then jettison the other two. Would you rather have a glass of wine than a slice of cake? Or do you opt for a slice of crusty Italian bread and forgo the Chianti and cannoli? You decide.

188. Be the last to pick up a fork.

Being the last to begin eating gives you time to get focused before you dig in. That is, to remember to eat slowly, to chew and taste your food, and to practice mindful eating in general.

Turn your wait into a game. Watch the way the others in your party hold their forks. See who gets spinach on his teeth.

189. Masquerade as a vegetarian.

If you're a meat eater, play a game when you dine out: See if you can order only meatless fare, such as salads, steamed vegetables, pasta with meatless sauce, and so on. Just make sure your selections are prepared without butter, cream, or cheese, which would send their calorie counts soaring.

Tools for High-Risk Situations: Navigating the Rough Spots

HOLIDAYS: CELEBRATION WITHOUT TEMPTATION

190. Bake nonedibles.

If you love to bake during the holidays, choose recipes you can't eat. Make fancy gingerbread men for the tree or a just-for-show gingerbread house. You can also surf the Web for recipes for pet treats or try bread-dough projects such as picture frames and magnets that you can decorate and give as gifts.

191. Gift wrap goodies—fast.

If you do choose to bake for family and friends, immediately wrap and tag the goodies. You won't be able to get at them.

192. Think beyond cookies.

This year, consider making healthy homemade gifts, such as herb-infused vinegars or salsas. Why make baked goods when you know you'll be tempted to sample them—and that the recipients will be struggling with holiday overeating, too?

193. Foil leftovers.

Your refrigerator will likely be groaning with leftovers the day after Christmas, Hanukkah, or New Year's. To distance yourself from the remains of your holiday meal, give them away or throw them out. Or plan a postholiday activity such as a trip to a museum with a friend, a long winter's walk in the woods, or a massage . . . something that's special and can divert your mind (and mouth) from the leftovers.

194. Make a must-have list.

When you make out your gift list, make yourself a food list: Write down all those tempting treats that usually wreak havoc on your eating program. Then select the five "musts": maybe your sister's irresistible chocolate-nut fudge or the creamy lobster Newburg that you look forward to each New Year's Eve. Making this list of tasty "allowables" fights the sense of deprivation that can lead to overeating. Looking forward to these special treats can also help you avoid food transgressions in between enjoying your "must-haves."

195. Swing into the holidays.

Before Thanksgiving, join a dance class, preferably one that builds on each week's lesson so you won't be tempted to skip a week. Swing dancing, tango, flamenco, ballroom . . . take your pick. Practice faithfully and you'll be in dazzling form by New Year's Eve.

196. Plan for the postvacation letdown.

As hard as it is not to overeat while on vacation, we don't often realize how hard it is not to overeat when we get home. After all, we're still on "vacation time," dreading the return of our everyday grind.

So before you leave on vacation, freeze some low-calorie meals (or stock up on healthy low-calorie entrées). That way, you don't have the work of deciding what to eat and then having to cook it. And because you have healthy food on hand, you won't be tempted to order out or go through a fast-food drive-thru.

NIGHT AND WEEKEND EATING: SUBDUE IT WITH STRUCTURE

197. Pull the old switcheroo.

Sometimes, our urge to eat coincides with our schedules or habits. Perhaps you go right into the kitchen when you get home from work for a slice of cheese or a handful of pretzels before you start dinner. Or maybe you're a night owl whose prime eating time is after 11:00 P.M.

See if your problem eating behaviors coincide with your schedule or habits. If you see a connection, modify them. Here are some examples of what I mean.

■ For after-work eaters: Don't go right into the kitchen when you come home from work. Go into the family room and switch on the evening news or go to the bathroom to brush your teeth, wash your face, or take a shower or bath.

■ If you play an instrument or work out: Switch your practice or workout time to the time when you would normally eat.

■ For late-night eaters: Create a bedtime schedule. You might bathe at a certain time, followed by a period of reading, followed by lights-out time. Then shorten the schedule by 15 minutes each night. Eventually, you may be able to fall asleep an hour earlier, which will shorten your overeating time. Caveat: Don't make TV a part of your schedule. You may continue to watch past your bedtime.

198. Try some night moves.

If you habitually raid the refrigerator when the sun goes down, get out of the house. One caveat: Food is everywhere, so you can't go just anywhere, especially not to the movies or to one of those mega bookstores that serve pastry and zillion-calorie coffee drinks. Three suggestions:

1. Buy tickets to a community play or musical. (You can't eat at a play like you can at the movies.)

2. Take a class at a local college. You'll improve your mind while you whittle your body.

3. Volunteer your time. Teach an adult to read, mentor a high-risk child, solicit donations for your local public radio or TV station.

199. Drop and do 10.

Before you pry open that tub of ice cream, do 10 situps or pushups. Distracting yourself with something physical can put you back in touch with your body—and your motivation.

200. Weekend eater? Try the two-meal tool.

On Saturdays and Sundays, many of us eat breakfast and lunch later than usual. At the same time, these meals are often bigger. Have just two meals—breakfast and dinner—and you'll save yourself a lump sum of calories. If you get hungry in between, have a small, nutritious snack.

201. Make weekend eating special.

If the two-meal tool works for you, make both of those meals an event by planning them during the week. Decide what healthy low-calorie fare is on your personal menu. Then make a list (always make a list) and buy your provisions. Go to the greengrocer and choose plump, delectable, farm-fresh fruits and vegetables or explore that upscale market you've been wanting to try.

202. Plan your splurges.

While you enjoy a Friday or Saturday night out, remember this: Letting loose is not letting go.

Plan your splurges by saving, say, 300 calories the day before your blowout. If your splurge ends up being more than you'd planned, analyze what went wrong. Did you have one too many alcoholic beverages, so your restraint went out the window? Did you let a friend talk you into ordering a high-calorie item "just this once"? Then eliminate the problem the next time you splurge.

203. Sweat out Saturdays and Sundays.

Weekends are a great time to get physical. For inspiration, see the Move Tools chapter.

OVEREATING: KEEP LITTLE SLIPS FROM SNOWBALLING

204. Corral those unplanned calories.

You have your whole eating day planned. Then bam! Your boss asks you to lunch and picks a pizza joint. Or you thought you'd be eating dinner at home but are persuaded to join your colleagues for an after-work get-together. Before you know it, you've eaten hundreds more calories than you'd planned—and you feel frustrated and guilty.

But don't "awfulize." Just use this tool to react *immediately* to a single bout of overeating. If you don't confront and react to one overeating event, it's likely you'll go on to another . . . and another. But if you face up to those extra calories fast, you'll be less likely to see them show up on the scale.

Before you use this tool, choose several low-calorie meals that have well-defined calorie counts. You'll use these meals to replace your usual meal, thereby compensating for those excess calories. Your meals might consist of a meal replacement, such as a liquid meal drink, or a protein bar or your favorite frozen diet dinners.

To put this tool to work for you:

1. Calculate your daily calories and analyze how you spread them throughout your day. For example, if you eat 1,800 calories per day, maybe you consume 250 for breakfast, 450 for lunch, 100 for a snack, and 1,000 for dinner.

2. Calculate the "surprise calories" you just ate. For example, if you spent the afternoon at the mall with a friend and had a large soft pretzel with mustard, look it up in your calorie counter.

3. Soft pretzels usually weigh about 7 ounces and pack about 500 calories. To compensate, you'll have to eat 500 calories less. But you can divvy those calories any way you want. If you want to compensate right away, you could "spend" 500 calories on dinner instead of the usual 1,000. End of problem. If you'd rather eat a heartier dinner, you could spend 700 calories (saving 300 calories), have a 150-calorie breakfast the next day (saving another 100 calories), and opt for a 350-calorie lunch (saving another 100 calories).

205. Cleanse your palate.

To stop a bout of overeating in its tracks, try this: Switch to an entirely different food. Let's say that, before you realize what you're doing, you eat half a bag of potato chips. You might as well finish them off, right? Wrong. Close the bag. Then cleanse your palate by eating a tomato or a small bunch of grapes. Eating something healthy gives you an opportunity to break away from the junk.

206. Munch in front of the mirror.

Buy a medium-size stand-up mirror and place it on the dining-room table when you eat. True, this tool is a bit over the top, and you may want to use it only when you're alone. But when you confront your mirror image in the midst of a chow-down, you may think twice about what—and how much—you eat.

TEMPTATION BLASTERS: STAY STRONG AND SAY NO

207. Shop on a full stomach.

Buy groceries when you're stomach's rumbling and you're likely to arrive home with high-calorie treats that you would have ignored had you not been hungry. Not to mention a significantly higher grocery bill.

208. Shop the outside aisles.

When you shop, keep to the perimeter of the store. Most supermarkets situate staples such as produce, meat, and dairy along the walls. Avoid the center aisles, which tend to be filled with the sweets and heavily processed foods.

209. Shop with a list. Always.

You'll know exactly what you need and what aisles to travel to get it. In fact, you should write an aisle-by-aisle list so your eyes—and willpower—don't waver.

210. Chew gum while you cook.

This tool is for those of us with Stovetop Syndrome—those of us who can't stand at the stove without "correcting the seasoning" or "testing" the pasta. I've found that my clients with Stovetop Syndrome stop nibbling if they chew sugarless gum as they cook. This gives their jaws the workout they need, without the extra calories they don't. Plus, if you do succumb to a nibble, you'll find that the taste of meat loaf or chili tends to clash with the flavor of cinnamon gum.

211. Blow bubbles in the face of temptation.

Start carrying sugarless chewing gum in your pocket or purse. Pop a stick into your mouth when you find yourself faced with "surprise food." While others eat, you can give your jaws a workout, too.

"UNLESS YOU TREAT YOURSELF, YOU'LL FEEL DEPRIVED"

There was a time when avid cook Meryl Collyns stood over her stove, spoon in hand, and tasted her creations. One taste led to another. And another. But that was then and this is now. For Collyns, cooking is still a passion but frequent tasting is a thing of the past.

"Cathy taught me to pop a Tic-Tac or piece of gum in my mouth while I cook," says Collyns, a nurse manager who shed 30 pounds and kept the weight off for 2 years. "With a Tic-Tac in your mouth, you won't taste your food because of the minty taste."

Collyns, a mother of two girls, once would finish her children's dinner, but she's kicked that habit, too. Now she places her daughters' leftovers into plastic containers that they take to school the next day. "Now I can't go back into the kitchen to nibble," Collyns says, laughing. "It's their lunch I'd be raiding. If food's going for my kids, I wouldn't dare eat it."

Even with a demanding schedule and long days as a nurse manager in obstetrics at a major hospital, Collyns takes the time to write down every morsel that goes into her mouth. If she takes two bites of a Three Musketeers Bar, Collyns dutifully records it. "A food diary not only keeps things in perspective,

Eventually, you'll automatically reach for a stick of gum during birthday parties at work, at the movies, and in front of the TV as your partner crunches away on chips.

212. When you feel shaky, stick to "safe foods."

When you feel like you want to overeat, pick a nutritious, low-calorie food to "binge" on. Wedge after wedge of fresh melon, enough salad for 22 people dressed with balsamic vinegar, or crispy fresh yellow, orange, and red peppers. Although you will have overeaten, you won't have the

it reinforces when you've had a good week," Collyns says. "And it shows you if you've had a not-so-great week." Another bonus, according to Collyns: Food diaries help a dieter track whether she's eating enough fruits and vegetables and an overall balanced diet.

Collyns is convinced she lost weight and keeps it off because she never denied herself the foods she loves but kept the portions reasonable. To treat herself, Collyns might sit down to one-third or one-half of a cannoli, an Italian pastry, with a cup of coffee. When she travels to England, where her husband was raised, Collyns delights in the British custom of tea but limits herself simply to a cucumber sandwich.

"Unless you treat yourself, you'll feel deprived," Collyns says. Two other tools in her weight-loss kit: Collyns doesn't sit too close to the table, so she must lean in to take bites, making gobbling less likely. Exercise is another staple. Collyns rises most mornings before her daughters rise to walk the treadmill. "Working out gives a mother some time to herself," Collyns says. "I'm doing a little something for me."

same feelings of guilt afterward. And it will be easier to get back on track the next meal.

213. Avoid drive-by eating.

We often eat in the car to keep ourselves entertained or awake—or simply because no one will know. But like eating while reading or watching TV, dashboard dining is "distracted eating." If you want to eat, stop the car first.

Part 3

YOUR TOP 40 DIET DANGER ZONES—SOLVED

Danger-Zone Basics

When it comes to weight loss, all of us have an Achilles heel—a specific situation or situations that can derail our program and undermine our good intentions.

I call these situations Diet Danger Zones. Their treachery—and power—is rooted in the fact that we often don't realize they exist or think we can overcome them with willpower alone. But if we can't or won't confront them, they can doom our weight-loss or weight-maintenance program to failure.

Sounds bleak, right? And yet, identifying our Diet Danger Zones can put us on the path to permanent weight loss, because once we can pinpoint our weak spots, we can begin to solve them.

We may never completely eradicate our Diet Danger Zones. (It's not likely that we'll ever become indifferent to chocolate!) But we *can* learn how to keep them from blindsiding our weight-loss efforts time and again.

There are as many Diet Danger Zones as there are dieters. But I've identified a core group of these trouble spots, and chances are you'll find yours among them. This section of the book lays out the 40 most common Diet Danger Zones, based on what I've seen in my years of helping thousands of people lose weight and keep it off.

Scan each Diet Danger Zone. Zero in on those that speak to you. You'll find simple, practical ways to whip each.

But that's just for starters. Turn to the numbers that run along the top right-hand side of each Diet Danger Zone. These are what I call "prescriptions"—specific tools that I believe can help you outwit a particular Diet Danger Zone most successfully.

If you'd rather, simply identify your Diet Danger Zones, then browse through the tools. You'll find tools that can help you plan and control your intake of calories, change self-destructive behaviors, become more active, or simply help you think more positively about yourself, your body, and your weight.

But that's not the end of your weight-loss journey—or the utility of this book. Often, our Diet Danger Zones change as our lifestyle and habits change. As we master one, another takes its place.

Here's one example. I once had a client who'd conquered her two biggest Diet Danger Zones: eating too much take-out food and blowing off exercise. Even so, she acquired a third: after-dinner snacking. She'd recently moved in with a man whose eating habits resembled those of a 7-year-old. Those handfuls of sugared cereal and heaping spoonfuls of peanut butter caused her to regain some of the weight she'd recently lost. Luckily, she was able to spot and get help for this new Diet Danger Zone before it became an ingrained behavior.

This story illustrates a key point: The cornerstone of successful weight loss is successful problem solving. You must search—hard—for answers to some tough questions. How, when, and why are you likely to overeat? What are you willing to do about it, and what aren't you? And how, specifically, will you do what you need to do to lose weight or keep it off?

If you're ready to start searching, your answers begin here.

You're tired.

Day or night, many of us reach for food when rest is what our bodies truly hunger for. Women are especially vulnerable to "fatigue eating": If you're the average woman, you sleep 6 hours and 41 minutes during the workweek, far less than the recommended 8 hours. We eat in a misguided attempt to keep our eyes open!

The obvious solution to fatigue eating? Get some sleep! You'll not only get the rest you need but also be less likely to end up rooting in the fridge during Leno or Letterman.

To ease your mind and body into an earlier bedtime, it's helpful to create a new evening routine. Some ideas:

- If you're frequently stressed when you arrive home from work, unwind before bed with a warm bath. Then indulge in a preslumber cup of chamomile tea.

- If you often take work home and nibble while you work far into the night, stock up on baby carrots. Crunch to your heart's content but put away your work an hour before you're ready to snooze. Then decompress with a warm soak or some light reading.

Fatigue eating hits in the afternoon, too. You may know it as the dreaded midafternoon slump. To fight it:

- Take an energy break. Get up from your desk and touch your toes 10 times or take a brisk jaunt around the office or up and down the stairs.

- If you're truly hungry, eat a small snack that complements the nutritional picture of your day. For example, if you want to consume more calcium, opt for a carton of low-fat yogurt. Choose a piece of fruit if you're on a low-fat plan or a small wedge of cheese if you're on a low-carbohydrate program.

DANGER ZONE #2 | TOOLS: 53, 63, 108, 109, 113, 166

You're angry.

Whether it's your boss, kid, partner, or the guy behind the counter at the department of motor vehicles that made your blood boil, anger and food are an explosive combination, akin to throwing kerosene on a fire. While I'm not a therapist, I've found that people who can't or won't express their anger tend to silence it with food. Unfortunately, the relief they find by avoiding their angry feelings is temporary. But the weight can stick around a long, long time.

Only you can decide whether unexpressed anger may be behind your inability to lose weight or maintain that weight loss. You may want to explore ways to let that ire out, whether by starting an anger journal, taking an assertiveness-training class, or even seeking therapy. In the meantime, here are some ways to stop "feeding" your anger.

- Use words—not food—to express your anger. Write a letter to the person who angered you. Really let him have it! When you're done, burn the letter. There. Don't you feel better?

- Exercise your anger out. If at all possible, take a brisk 10-minute walk. It will keep you at a safe distance from the cookies in your pantry or the vending machine at work.

- Establish the texture of the food you want. If you tend to reach for crunchy foods (such as chips) when you're angry, opt for foods that offer crunch without weighty consequences (such as Cheerios or air-popped popcorn).

- When we're angry, we tend to eat while standing. If you must eat, do it as a guest in your home would: sitting at the dining-room table and using a plate and utensils. Sitting gives you a sense of control.

You're bored.

When your lack of anything better to do threatens to turn your kitchen into one big Diet Danger Zone, find something—anything—to do. Fast. Try these suggestions.

▪ Now, before the next bout of boredom eating hits, figure out when you usually experience this problem. Then devise and write out a plan of attack. Here's a sample.

When boredom eating typically takes place: On weekend days from about 2:00 to 5:00 P.M.

Plan: Go for a 60-minute walk or go to the gym.

When: Saturday and Sunday from 2:00 to 3:00 P.M.

Where: High-school track in good weather, mall in bad weather.

With whom: A friend, colleague, or neighbor.

With a plan in place, you'll be much less likely to be in the kitchen at 2:30 on a Saturday afternoon with a squeeze bottle of chocolate syrup in one hand and a spoon in the other.

▪ On an index card, make a list of 10 things to do when you have "nothing" to do. A sample list might include: read a book, write a letter, go to the park, go to the craft store or bookstore, start a jigsaw puzzle, call a friend, play solitaire, swing on your child's swing set, whatever. When you have nothing to do and you find yourself in the kitchen, pick something from the list and do it. Don't think about it. Just do it. Some folks laminate a few cards and stick one on their refrigerator and one on their pantry or cupboard door.

▪ If you just can't get out the door, make yourself a huge salad. Like enough for 22 people. Every time you open the refrigerator door, eat a few forkfuls.

DANGER ZONE #4

You're stressed.

You've got a demanding job, a demanding family, demanding friends, and a boatload of stress. And you're not alone, especially if you're a woman. A recent survey found that 8 percent of women report they feel stress at the end of every day; 21 percent feel it almost every day; and 29 percent once or twice a week.

Many of us attempt to soothe our stress with food. While eating may temporarily reduce our stress, it will often increase it in the long run, especially if we berate ourselves for putting on weight.

Using food to cope with stress is a habit that we develop, so it's a habit we can change. The next time you're about to lose it, try these suggestions.

- If at all possible, take a 20-minute break. If you're at home, slap on a facial mask, do your nails, or get into bed and read for a bit.

- Listen to soothing music.

- Exhale slowly and relax your muscles as you do so. As you exhale, say silently, "I feel tension flowing out of my body." Do this five or six times and you'll become more relaxed.

- Turn to a hobby. Busy hands are less likely to feed you. Take up needlework. Get out in the garden. Put together jigsaw puzzles. Log on to an online gaming site for a rousing round of Scrabble.

DANGER ZONE #5

TOOLS: 29, 96, 112, 135, 176, 186

You're coping with a major stressor such as a career change, caring for an aging parent, or separation or divorce.

Stress caused by an ongoing major change or trauma can make us feel out of control. And when we feel that our lives are in a tailspin, food can become a major—perhaps only—source of comfort.

But in times of trouble, we must make a supreme effort to care for ourselves and to cut ourselves a break. Here are some ways to do that.

- Reach out. Unburdening yourself to a trusted friend, relative, or member of the clergy can significantly reduce your stress.

- Escape—temporarily. Go to a movie. Visit a museum. If you can, take a weekend road trip with a friend. It will give you a much-needed boost.

- Reward yourself regularly. Starting today, reward yourself with little things that make you feel good. Treat yourself to a bubble bath, buy the hardcover edition of a book, call an old friend long-distance, buy yourself flowers, picnic in the park on your lunch hour. Or do something you wouldn't ordinarily do, such as go to the theater or a museum.

- Do a relaxation exercise daily. Good ones include visualization (imagining a soothing, restful scene), deep muscle relaxation (tensing and relaxing muscle fibers), meditation, and deep breathing.

DANGER ZONE #6

TOOLS: 48, 51, 55, 107, 157, 202

You have a craving.

You're well into your weight-loss program and you feel great. But trust me. There will come a time when you hear Oreos or a pint of Häagen-Dazs call your name. And how you answer that call just might make or break your success at weight loss and maintenance.

The key is to change the way you think about cravings. Don't try to resist them. *Manage* them. When you accept them—even expect them—they lose their power. Here's how not to let a craving derail your progress.

- Sip a glass of water. Sometimes we mistake dehydration for hunger or cravings.

- Ride the wave of your craving. A wave in the ocean gathers, peaks, and then subsides. A craving works much the same way—if you don't give in to it. Wait for 20 minutes to see if your craving diminishes.

- Use the Five Ds. See Diet Danger Zone #7.

- Don't skip meals. It's harder to resist a craving for a fast-food super-size meal at dinner when you haven't eaten breakfast or lunch.

- Pinpoint your craving. If only Häagen-Dazs chocolate-chip ice cream will do, then have it. But before you do, plan how you will control your portion size. You might throw on your coat, grab a spoon from home, buy a pint, eat half, and throw the other half away in the store parking lot.

You feel a binge coming on.

First, a clarification: I use the word "binge" here because so many people use it as a synonym for overeating. But clinically, a "binge" is not eating 10 cookies instead of 1 or eating a huge dinner. It's consuming massive amounts of food in a short period of time at least twice a week for at least 6 months, with accompanying feelings of guilt and shame.

Still, an episode of overeating can leave you frustrated and depressed enough to abandon your weight-loss or maintenance program—which makes it a powerful Diet Danger Zone indeed.

The best way to avoid a binge? Don't set yourself up for one. Practice and use stress-management techniques, take time to nurture yourself the way you would others, and learn to recognize your own personal "warning signs" of an impending binge. These tips can help.

- HALT! Alcoholics Anonymous has a wonderful saying that helps remind its members to take care of themselves: "Never get too Hungry, Angry, Lonely, or Tired." The idea is that people are more likely to pick up a drink if they're in any of these conditions—and it's frequently true of overeaters, too. Adopting this slogan may help you avoid physical and emotional Danger Zones that can trigger a binge.

- Use the Five Ds. This technique can help you stop and think about what you're about to do when the chips or the peanut-butter jar is in your hand.

Determine what's going on. Ask yourself, "Why do I want to eat so badly right now?"

Delay your response. Don't immediately give in to your urge to eat. If you stall long enough, the craving may well pass.

Distract yourself for at least 10 minutes.

Distance yourself from temptation. At home, throw your binge food down the disposal or cover it with cayenne pepper. (Hey, whatever keeps you from picking it out of the trash.)

Decide how you'll handle the situation. Will you stop eating or continue? If you decide to keep going, at least you'll have thought about your behavior, understand why you're engaging in it, and accept the consequences.

■ Formally forgive yourself. Fight the voice inside your head that whispers you're a glutton with no willpower. Instead, tell yourself: "Yes, I slipped—and I hereby forgive myself."

■ As soon as you can after the binge, reconstruct the entire episode—on paper. Write exactly what led to the binge and the strategies you might have used to stop it. The act of analyzing your binge may calm you, making you more receptive to what went wrong, which makes it easier to use strategies to help you avoid those circumstances next time.

■ No matter what time of day your overeating occurs and no matter how guilty or disgusted you may feel, eat your next scheduled meal. Immediately resuming your normal eating routine can help fight off the "what the heck, I've blown it" attitude that may have undermined your past weight-loss attempts.

DANGER ZONE #8   TOOLS: 53, 63, 82, 119, 120

After your workout, you raid the refrigerator.

Why are some of us so ravenous after a workout? Darned if I know. The results of more than 100 studies show that if you burn, say, 300 calories exercising, you won't compensate for them by eating more, especially if you're overweight. (Normal-weight folks do tend to compensate, which makes sense since their weight remains stable.)

Still, many of my clients insist they're ready to gnaw the veneer off their kitchen cupboards after a good hard workout. If this sounds like you, these suggestions can help you get through the postworkout food blowout. Just remember: Control the portion size before you put even one morsel into your mouth.

- Drink lots of water, both during and after your workout. Your "hunger" may actually be thirst.

- If you exercise during the day, have a snack 45 minutes to an hour before your workout. Good bets: one slice of whole grain bread with 1 tablespoon of peanut butter, one piece of fruit, or a small box of raisins.

- If that doesn't work, eat your snack *after* your workout rather than before. It may help keep you from overeating at your next meal.

- If you exercise after work and you arrive home famished, tuck a small snack into your gym bag to tide you over.

Your job requires you to eat on the run.

Whether you're a sales rep with clients all over the region, a paramedic who regularly downs grab-and-go meals, or a high-powered type who logs serious behind-the-wheel time rushing to meeting to conference to airport, you probably choke down your fair share of fast-food fare, convenience-store offerings, and what passes for food in vending machines. Your mealtimes are at the mercy of your schedule and whatever food is available, wherever you happen to be. And when you're trying to shed pounds or keep lost pounds lost, that loss of control—and choice—puts you squarely in the Diet Danger Zone.

But it doesn't have to. The key is to exert the control you *do* have into your otherwise chaotic schedule. But to wrest back that control, you have to do some troubleshooting. Ask yourself these questions:

- Although I'm frequently on the fly, am I usually in the same area? Might I search out restaurants that offer healthy, low-calorie fare or supermarkets along my route that offer a make-it-yourself salad bar?

- Could I pack and carry my own proportioned meals to eat on plane or train trips or between clients? (It's generally a bad idea to eat in the car, but this solution may be your best bet.)

- If I'm typically on the run in the morning, could I eat a larger breakfast to tide me over until lunch? If I'm on the go all day, could I pack one or two meals rather than stop at a fast-food joint or convenience store? In situations like these, you might opt for a meal-replacement bar (sold in most convenience stores). The caveat: You really do have to consider it a meal.

- Think of three meals you could get virtually anywhere, from a convenience store to an airport: say, a turkey sandwich (no cheese or mayo), a meal-replacement bar, or a salad or soup and a roll. Those will be your default meals when there's nothing even remotely healthful to be found.

DANGER ZONE #10

TOOLS: 12, 74, 75, 83, 141, 188

You're facing a business lunch or dinner.

So there's this very important client who could award a $250,000 contract to your firm. Go ahead, max out your corporate credit card. Take him or her to the best restaurant in town. But don't fool yourself: There's no reason you must eat or drink yourself into oblivion to seal the deal. Whether you're the winer and diner or the wined and dined, you *can* avoid this Diet Danger Zone. Some advice:

- The day before your meeting, call the restaurant and ask them to recommend a few low-fat, low-calorie dishes. Most will be glad to help, and some may even accommodate special requests.

- As you enter the dining room, tell yourself you're there first to conduct business and secondarily to eat. We often associate restaurant meals with pleasure and stress reduction. So reminding yourself that you're eating for business, not pleasure, may strengthen your resolve to opt for lighter fare.

- Pull a no-brainer and order the "executive's special": A salad (low-fat dressing on the side), grilled poultry or fish (minus the fatty sauces), a steamed vegetable, and a low-calorie beverage.

- Imagine yourself trying to cut a deal after a heavy meal and a couple of glasses of Chardonnay.

DANGER ZONE #11 TOOLS: 29, 37, 97, 125, 139, 151, 160

You work at home . . . and the refrigerator beckons.

When you work at home, there's no boundary of time or space to define mealtime. You can eat breakfast at 5:00 A.M. or at 10:45. Any room in the house can be your cafeteria. And when you can't sit at your desk another minute, it's all too easy to wander into the kitchen.

- One of the best ways to work and eat at home is to define your "eating zone." Make it a policy to eat in one place during work hours: at the table, sitting down, using a plate and utensils.

- Don't combine work with meals. If you want to eat lunch, stop working. But don't work and eat at the same time, in the same place.

- Have your first meal of the day later in the day. It's often easier to delay eating than to stop eating.

- Keep a bottle of water or a thermos of coffee or tea on your desk. That will keep you from going into the kitchen for a drink—and mindless in-front-of-the-refrigerator nibbling.

- Don't eat at home during the day at all, even for lunch. Go out at midday for a short walk and a meal.

The holiday season has begun.

The weeks from Thanksgiving through New Year's Day are filled with warm family gatherings, cheery get-togethers with friends and colleagues . . . and lots of high-calorie, high-fat treats. The suggestions below can help you navigate this Diet Danger Zone—and spare your waistline.

- Come the holidays, don't skip breakfast or lunch. You'll just overeat at the company party or nosh Christmas cookies and candy at the office in the midafternoon.

- As much as you love eggnog, pass it up—and limit yourself to one alcoholic beverage. They're loaded with calories.

- Be selective. Eat the things you really love—a small serving of mashed potatoes, a thin sliver of pecan pie—and ignore the not-so-thrilling stuff.

- Chew gum at holiday events where food will be served. It will give you something to do with your mouth other than eat.

- At a buffet, scrutinize the foods before you put them on your plate. Take a serving-spoon size of the foods you really want and smaller portions of the foods you just want to taste.

- If you'll be a guest at someone's home, volunteer to bring a fruit salad or raw veggie plate. You'll know that there will be at least one thing you can feel good about nibbling.

DANGER ZONE #13 | TOOLS: 42, 98, 108, 121, 179, 188

There's a food pusher in your life.

It could be your mother, your friends, or, God help you, even your partner. You know the drill: "You'll get sick if you don't eat." "One little piece won't hurt you." And they can be hard to argue with. If they're at the kitchen table with a slice of cheesecake, you know you'll be served a slice whether you want it or not.

While food pushers don't always harbor evil intent, it's entirely possible that the one in your life doesn't want you to lose weight or maintain your weight loss. No matter. Because it's up to you to learn to deflect the food pushers—and if you can't, to avoid them as much as possible. These tactics can help.

- If you regularly meet for dinner or drinks with a friend or a group of colleagues, suggest an activity in which food isn't the main attraction. They may enjoy a night at the bowling lane, the movies, or the karaoke bar. And if they won't, find friends who will.

- If you suspect the food pushers want to see you fail, kill them with kindness. Say, "Boy, that pizza looks great. But I'm just not hungry right now." Or "Your cinnamon buns are always delicious. But I'm trying not to eat sugar." Be assertive without being aggressive, be polite but stand firm. When you're alone, practice saying no—in front of the mirror, if necessary.

- Consider that they may feel uncomfortable eating in front of you. If you feel that's the case, tell them that you're just fine and that they should enjoy their pie and coffee or whatever.

- Remember this: As long as you're in control of your own behavior, nobody and nothing can sway you from your weight-loss or weight-maintenance program. Come your kids' junk food or a colleague's birthday cake, you can handle the food pushers and the temptation to cheat they serve up.

Your partner says he "likes you just the way you are."

This is one of the toughest Diet Danger Zones there is, because it's hard to discern his motives. He could be sincere. Or he could be threatened by your weight loss. He may even fear that if you become more attractive, you may stray.

■ Decide how your partner could most help. (He may want to help but is unsure of how.) Do you want compliments and active encouragement? His help with grocery shopping or cooking? Would you like him to work out with you or watch the kids or start supper while you exercise? Also, how do you want him to react if you slip, lose or gain weight, or dine out?

■ In a quiet, relaxed moment, talk honestly with your partner. Only you will know the right words. But you might say something along the lines of "I know you say you like me as I am. But losing weight (or keeping it off) is really important to me, and I'd like to talk about how you might help me."

■ If your spouse responds positively, hash out the details of exactly how he is willing to help. Both of you should feel free to make your desires known, but neither should expect to get everything you want.

■ If your partner is less than supportive, try different ways to work around him to make the environment safer. For example, you might make two vegetables instead of one (make them vegetables you especially love) and fill your plate. Or have your partner help you with the dishes so you can't pick at leftovers.

You eat as you cook . . . and then again at the table.

If you nibble at the stove and then follow it up with a full-size meal, you may be packing away double the calories you think you are! These suggestions can help you break what I call "Stovetop Syndrome."

- Chew sugarless gum as you cook. This gives your jaws the workout they need, without the extra calories you don't.

- Keep a water bottle on the counter as you cook. Train yourself to take a sip of water every time you want to taste-test. If you cook each night, consider setting a goal: to drink 1 liter of water by the time you're finished preparing the evening meal.

- Allow yourself to taste your creation once—just before you serve it, to correct the seasoning.

You're at a big celebration . . . and when you're happy, you eat.

In a situation like this, your impulse is to hide your head in the sand. It's a celebration, right? No worries, no cares, and no self-restraint, either. If you don't care about sticking to your program in this situation, you may feel sorry later. Here's how to celebrate without guilt.

- Preplan. Decide those situations in which you're going to let go and those in which you're going to follow your plan. Then actually write down your plan. "I'm going to sit down and order a vodka tonic. I'm going to keep my chair away from the table so I don't automatically reach for food. I am going to order _____."

- Tell someone else to order for you. Relay your request the day before, if possible.

- Order what you really want to *taste*—say, the lobster tail. And order the lowest-calorie courses when it doesn't matter. For example, if you don't much like vegetables, order them steamed.

- Don't drink an alcoholic beverage until your food arrives. Alcohol may stimulate your appetite.

You eat when you read or watch television.

One day, one of my clients, following the Weight Watchers program, decided to have a snack—a few chips. After she converted the number of fat grams and calories to points, she found she could have 12 chips. She did the math but still ended up munching handfuls of chips at a time.

Suddenly, she felt a decidedly unchiplike object in her mouth. She fished it out. It was a coupon, sealed in protective wrap.

Talk about mindless eating.

As my client found, when we eat mindlessly, we have little or no awareness of what food actually tastes like, let alone how much of it we eat. The most obvious and successful solution to this Danger Zone is to eat at the dining-room table, bereft of book or remote control.

But what if you *like* eating while you read or watch TV so much that you're not willing to give it up? That's when it's time to try the tips below.

- Pick one low-calorie food that you like and that you can eat a reasonably large portion of without exceeding your daily calorie allotment. Examples might include baby carrots with salsa or another raw vegetable, air-popped popcorn, or straw-berries. Place them in a bowl and eat with chopsticks. (That's right—even if you're eating popcorn.) The chopsticks will force you to pay attention to your food and also slow you down.

- Designate TV time or reading time as your time to make a dent in your daily water requirement.

- For TV watchers: Move the television. Or consider watching your favorite shows on the TV in your bedroom, if you have one (or on the TV the farthest away from the kitchen). If you later decide to have a snack, you'll have to travel to get it, which will make you more conscious of your decision to eat.

- For readers: Consider reading in a warm bath instead of on the couch or in your family room or bedroom. It's hard to munch mindlessly when you're trying to keep your reading material dry.

You're on a medication that stimulates your appetite.

This Danger Zone is a particularly difficult one because the medicine is likely making you feel better, even if it leaves you continually ravenous. It may be possible for your doctor to substitute another medication for the one that's stimulating your appetite or making you gain weight. If that's not an option, you'll need to be especially vigilant about what you put in your mouth. These suggestions can help.

- Eat more often. Just eat smaller portions. The easiest way to do this is to divide your meal into threes. Eat your meat and vegetable first. Two hours later, eat your salad. Two hours after that, eat your potato.

- Add more fiber or protein to your diet. Both tend to be filling. Experiment to see which one leaves you more satisfied.

- Eat lower-calorie foods as "filler," then add small amounts of your favorite foods. (Just don't have too many of them lying around the house!)

DANGER ZONE #19

TOOLS: 27, 35, 36, 45, 102, 107, 113, 135, 150, 159, 168

You've been "good," but the scale says you've gained 2 pounds.

It's a contraption made of plastic, metal, and cheap springs and coils. But the Almighty Scale holds enormous power. When the number is right, we can almost hear a heavenly chorus. But when it's wrong, woe to us. It can shoot the whole day straight to heck—along with your diet and exercise program. But that's only if you let it. Here's how to strip the scale of its power.

- No matter how frustrated you are, keep the focus on your behavior, not on what the scale says. You know that your weight can fluctuate from day to day. Don't let a minor blip on the scale lead you toward a piece of chocolate cake or keep you out of the gym. Trust me: If you've been faithful to your diet and exercise program, the weight will come off.

- Keep a food diary. If you already are, make sure you're not fudging portion sizes or ignoring food you eat as you prepare meals. They can really add up, and you may be eating hundreds of calories more a day than you think you are. If you haven't yet started a food diary, turn to page 208 for information on how to begin.

- Lose the perfectionist attitude. As I wrote in the chapter Exchange Your FATitudes for FITitudes, thinking you have to "do" dieting perfectly or not at all is a FATitude that will ultimately sabotage your weight-loss goals. You didn't "fail"; you had a minor setback (or perhaps a normal fluctuation in weight). Don't fail yourself by seeking comfort at the fast-food drive-thru.

- Scrutinize your everyday schedule to see whether your life has changed in any way. Are you taking a new medication? Dining out more frequently or exercising less? If you keep a food diary, scour it for clues. If you don't keep one, start. You may find that you're eating more than you thought.

You've been on a plateau for 2 weeks now.

To many of us, this Diet Danger Zone is actually a special circle of hell on earth reserved for those trying to lose weight. But don't throw in the towel! Your plateau may be a simple case of water retention. The key: Don't sabotage yourself. These tips can help you hang in there through this maddening period.

■ Don't focus just on the numbers. Evaluate how you feel. Do you have more energy? Do you sleep better? Feel healthier? Even if the pounds aren't exactly peeling off, you're probably still reaping the benefits of eating less and moving more.

■ Increase the duration or intensity of your workout. Walk a little farther or a little faster. Also, if you haven't already, introduce weight training to your regimen. Lifting weights builds muscle, and muscle burns more calories than fat.

■ Study your journal. It can help you see if you may be going over your daily calorie or point allotment or help pinpoint other trouble spots. Look over your journal for the past 2 weeks and try to identify any negative patterns that may be the cause of your plateau.

■ Weigh and measure portions. Break out the measuring cups and spoons. See if you're suddenly eating larger portions of peanut butter, pasta, or salad dressing than you thought.

"TOOLS DO MAKE A DIFFERENCE"

Rosita Sarnoff lost 20 pounds slowly—over a period of 18 months. But she's kept them off. And in the weight-loss game, that spells success.

Sarnoff, a 58-year-old senior vice president of a residential real estate firm, believes in the power of tools. "They help break unhealthy eating patterns and encourage good ones. They also get your motivation going and keep it going. They really do make a difference."

Sarnoff often dines out: Her life is a whirl of cocktail parties, business lunches and dinners, and benefits. The tools that help her navigate the treacheries of social-event eating and expense-account dining can help anyone who eats out more often than in.

At cocktail parties, Sarnoff makes a choice: She either has hors d'oeuvres and no dinner or decides on dinner and skips the finger foods. She doesn't order an alcoholic beverage until her meal arrives. (Alcohol tends to loosen inhibitions, including those that tell you not to order dessert.) She won't dip into the bread basket until her main course arrives. "Usually, by the time my meal comes, I don't want the bread anyway," says Sarnoff.

Her most commonly used eating-out tool? "Don't eat anything white." Sarnoff limits her intake of starchy foods, such as potatoes, and those that consist primarily of refined carbohydrates, such as white bread and pasta.

Tools also help her master her primary Danger Zone: eating when she arrives home from work.

Before she leaves the office or upon arriving home, she has a small but healthy snack—a piece of cheese and an apple or a small container of yogurt. This tool alone—identifying her prime "snack time" and planning for it—keeps her from picking until dinnertime, which often arrives as late as 9:00 P.M.

But Sarnoff doesn't need tools to get in regular physical activity. Twice a week, under the watchful eye of her trainer, she does an hour-long strength-training and aerobic workout. On the weekends, she takes long walks.

While Sarnoff wants to lose another 10 pounds, she says that the key to success is modifying the eating behaviors that put on the weight in the first place. And although changing those behaviors can take time, she knows the rewards of doing so can last a lifetime.

You're on vacation and can't resist the local fare.

Ah, vacations. Freedom from the office. Freedom from routine. And, unfortunately, freedom from our weight-loss or weight-maintenance programs. Yes, vacations are a challenge. But with a little planning, you'll enjoy your vacation without arriving home with "excess baggage."

- If your health and weight permit, take a more active vacation. Instead of spending a week lazing around a cabana in Mexico, pedal *une bicyclette* in Provence. You're bound to find an active vacation to fit your interest and budget.

- While car trips can be easy on the budget, they can be murder on healthy eating. Plan ahead: Pack a large cooler filled with ice water, diet drinks, whole grain crackers, low-fat yogurt, and a variety of sliced raw fruit and veggies. When your cooler is empty, find another grocery store and fill 'er up again.

- Whether you vacation in Europe or camp in the mountains, make a point to walk, hike, or bike each day, rather than simply climb into your car or the tour bus. If you're on a cruise, take a brisk walk or jog around the top deck.

- Designate one meal a day as your "indulgence" meal. If you savor a hefty serving of bread and cheese in Paris for lunch, opt for a modest dinner. Or choose fruit and fat-free yogurt or a bowl of cereal and fruit rather than the hotel's breakfast buffet.

- Sometimes, the most difficult part of a vacation is returning home. Before you leave, schedule two sessions with a personal trainer for the week you return home. If that's not an option, stock up on healthy frozen dinners so that you won't have to think about what to eat when you get home.

DANGER ZONE #22

Your family won't eat healthy fare, and you can't resist their goodies.

You say chicken stir-fry with broccoli and carrots over brown rice. They say meat loaf with gravy and mashed potatoes. Should you call the whole weight-loss thing off? No. It is possible to follow your diet plan despite feeding a family addicted to Little Debbie's cakes and BBQ potato chips. The whole family could use more healthy options to go with their chips. Try these.

- To help fill you up but not out, start your meal with tomato or vegetable soup, consommé, a salad drizzled with light dressing, or a piece of fruit.

- Don't add butter or margarine to veggies, potatoes, or grains when you cook them. Instead, let each family member add his or her own.

- Stop dining "family style," which covers the table with bowls and platters of food. It's harder to resist seconds. Instead, keep the food in the kitchen and make a plate for each family member. Bring *only* the plates to the table. Those who want seconds can go to the kitchen and help themselves.

- Designate a special cabinet for your family's snack foods, preferably a lower cabinet or a lower shelf on the pantry. If the chips and cookies are all in one place, you won't have to confront them—and the temptation to eat them—every time you reach for a rice cake or a bag of air-popped popcorn.

- Prepare the meals your family enjoys—with conditions. First, you'll make smaller portions. Second, you won't put the food on the table. They can refill their plates at the stove or countertop. Third, you'll make more vegetables. Fourth, they'll have to scrape their plates into the garbage and put the leftovers in the fridge, so you won't pick at the scraps.

You're newly in love ... and you're truly eating for two.

There's a natural connection between food and love. When we feed the ones we love or eat a meal together, we feel nurtured, just as we did when Mom served up fresh-baked cookies. And it's all too easy to stare into one another's eyes over untold candlelit dinners or cocoon on the couch with two spoons and a half-gallon of cookie-dough ice cream. If you face this Diet Danger Zone, you'll need to think more clearly about food's role in your life and in your relationship and then brainstorm to devise intimate activities that don't involve food. These suggestions can help.

- Ease up on dining out, even if it's his treat. Suggest a more active activity—perhaps an hour of in-line skating or bicycling in the park, a walk along the lake, or a night of bowling (minus the nachos and beer).

- When you cook him his favorite meals, add some of your favorite low-calorie, healthy foods, too. Or enjoy the meal you make for him with some creative variations. For example, you might have a 3-ounce portion of his Fred Flintstone–sized porterhouse, along with a baked potato (no butter) and the steamed asparagus you make for him, minus the hollandaise sauce. (Just don't snack on the leftovers later.)

- If you and he like to snuggle in front of the TV with a bag of chips, proffer a tray of raw vegetables with a fat-free dip instead. If he turns up his nose, crunch on the carrots yourself. At least you'll be crunching. Or better yet, change your eating behavior. Eat in only one room—the dining room.

- Keep his snack food in its own cupboard, away from your healthier fare. Teach him where the cupboard is. And then forget it exists.

You're so bored with your diet that you're ready to hold up a Hostess delivery truck.

No doubt about it: The same-old, same-old can get mighty boring, whether you're on your "old" diet—the gain-weight diet—or a newer low-carbohydrate or high-carbohydrate diet. Your boredom may be a sign that your program is too restrictive. Adding a bit of flexibility into your food choices may make your diet more bearable. Try these tips.

- Take back some of the foods you've eliminated from your diet. Take egg yolks, for example. So many of us make do with egg-white omelets. But a poached egg with the yolk can taste so rich and satisfying that you may not need a handful of chocolate kisses later. If you miss bacon, consider this: A bacon, lettuce, and tomato sandwich without mayo is only about 300 calories.

- Add, then take away. If you absolutely must have a slice of pizza or if you miss the ice cream you used to have every night after dinner, have it—but eat fewer calories at dinner.

You've fallen off your exercise plan, which makes you less careful about your diet.

There's a domino effect at play here. When you're not active, you don't take care of your body. You stop drinking water, eating your vegetables, parking your car in the space farthest away from the mall entrance. You're in a rut, waiting for a bolt of lightning to blast you out. Here's what to do.

- Even though you're not working out, feed your body as though you were. Drink that water, nibble on fresh raw vegetables, control your portion sizes, monitor your intake of fatty foods such as butter and cheese.

- If you can't or won't exercise, eat less. Reduce or cut out snacks and eat smaller portions at mealtimes.

- List on paper all the things you currently do to live a healthy life. Even if you're not exercising, you may find that you're eating well, monitoring your eating behavior, keeping a food diary, and thinking positively. This list helps you realize that all is not lost if you're not currently exercising.

- Hire a personal trainer once a week to boost your motivation.

You love to cook ... and want desperately to bake your legendary death by chocolate cake.

When you love to cook for family and friends, losing weight or maintaining that loss can be a tough proposition. But it may be possible for you to continue to create gourmet masterpieces without piling on the pounds. Here's how.

- Invest in a couple of low-fat cookbooks and throw your culinary passion into creating lighter, healthier fare. Experiment with exotic vegetables, noodles, whole grains, beans, seafood. Or simply figure out how to make your best-loved recipes less caloric. You might add something "exotic" such as dandelion greens to your salads or sauté grapes as a side dish for fish.

- Serve two low-calorie courses for every high-calorie one.

- Use big plates and small servings to add elegance to the meal—and to reduce the temptation to overeat.

- Invest in low-fat cooking tools. The essentials: a steamer, no-stick sauté pans, and a small, inexpensive food processor for chopping flavor enhancers such as garlic, onions, and fresh herbs.

- To lower the fat content of your baked goodies, replace some of the butter or oil with mashed or pureed fruit, such as bananas or dates. Substitute unsweetened cocoa for most of the unsweetened chocolate called for in a recipe. And use low-fat milk instead of cream or whole milk.

- Chew gum as you cook. You'll be less likely to taste-test, which can add up to hundreds of unwanted calories.

DANGER ZONE #27 TOOLS: 15, 17, 22, 23, 87, 125, 149, 202

You're a mall eater.

You just can't resist those whopper cinnamon buns, pizza, double lattes, or the nachos dripping with cheese. With all this temptation in one place, it can be hard to make the right choices at the mall. But with a little forethought, you can avoid those junk-food land mines.

- Eat before you go to the mall. If you're with friends who want to eat before or after they shop, bring a healthy snack, such as a bag of baby carrots or a piece of fruit. Or treat yourself to a cappuccino with fat-free milk. (No biscotti!)

- Carry a bottle of water. Mall air tends to be dry and can make you thirsty—and many of us reach for food when what we really need is water.

- Have a game plan before the sights and smells get the better of you. Walk past all the food stands first. Then decide what you really want.

- If you're with friends, split an item, like a small order of nachos or an order of fries. For a full meal, add a salad with dressing on the side. That way, you can enjoy what you love without overdoing it.

- Make smart choices: grilled, broiled, or baked chicken or fish sandwiches or wraps made with lean meats or veggies. If you want tuna salad, ask to see it first so you can make sure it's not loaded with high-fat mayo.

DANGER ZONE #28

You have Garbage Pail Syndrome . . . you eat the leftovers off your kids' plates.

If you think those few last forkfuls of your kids' TV dinner don't count, think again. The American Dietetic Association estimates that, by nibbling on leftovers at most dinners, you can add an additional 150 calories to your diet each day. That equals a pound a month! Here's how to stop the gain.

■ If you can't stand throwing away perfectly good food, serve your kids smaller portions. They can always ask for seconds.

■ If they're old enough (and they're almost always old enough!), have your kids scrape their plates into the garbage after their meal.

■ If they're too little to help, have your partner clear the dishes. (Once the danger's past, you can wash.)

■ Chew gum as you clear the table so you won't nibble off their plates.

■ Kids are notorious for leaving tons of leftovers. So when you eat in a restaurant, order whatever your kids want and tea for yourself. Then nibble off their plates and call it your meal.

You follow a low-fat diet and eat only low-fat snack foods, but you're gaining weight.

This Danger Zone is so common it's been given a name: Snackwell's Syndrome. These low-fat snacks may contain just a smidge of fat, but they're usually loaded with sugar and calories. While there's nothing intrinsically evil about low-fat baked goods or snacks, *fat-free* does not mean *calorie-free*. Here's how to treat the syndrome.

■ Think about snacks in a new light: They're not "free" foods but those that complete your nutritional requirements. Do you need more calcium, fiber, or fruit in your diet? Use your snacks to get them.

■ Outwit the temptation to eat straight from the box or bag. Divide the snack into 1-ounce portions and store them in plastic bags.

■ Better yet, buy single-portion low- or no-fat snacks, readily available at convenience stores.

■ If you have to store boxes of low-fat snack cakes, pastries, or doughnuts in your house, store them in the back of your highest kitchen cabinet. When you want some, measure out one serving and immediately put the rest away.

■ Try eating larger meals. Some of us have a tendency to reduce our meals to accommodate the extra calories we spend on snacks. The result? A snack and a meal look very, very similar. But a meal is necessary. A snack, depending on why you're having it, can be extraneous.

You can't get through a movie without an extra-large popcorn.

When we were kids, a jaunt to the movies wasn't complete without a stop at the concession stand for buttery popcorn or sugary treats. But taking in a flick doesn't have to mean letting out your seams. The obvious solution: Don't eat anything. But if that's not feasible, try the suggestions below.

- Take your own popcorn. There are lots of brands of low-fat, low-cal microwave popcorns. If you like sweets, tote a Tootsie Pop.

- Take a bottle of water so you won't have to go near the concession stand for refreshments.

- Consider buying your tickets in advance. When you pick them up at the box office, you can go straight into the theater without waiting in line, watching everyone else buy goodies.

- If all else fails and you can't resist the call of the concession stand: Choose licorice (fat- and calorie-wise, Twizzlers are your best bet). The portion size can be huge, so either buy a small package at a drugstore before the movie or throw away (or give away) most of the mammoth theater-size portion.

DANGER ZONE #31

TOOLS: 27, 62, 66, 86, 126, 160

From November 1 to March 31, your willpower goes south with the geese.

For would-be weight watchers, the foodfest that is the holiday season is a bad time. So are the dark, dreary months afterward. And where are we likely to spend them? In front of the refrigerator. While a *New England Journal of Medicine* study suggests that average-weight folks usually gain about 1 pound during the holidays, those of us who are already overweight are likely to gain an average of 5. Worse, we don't typically lose the weight we gain during the winter months. To help head off hibernation pounds, try the suggestions below.

■ Test-drive winter sports. Ever skied? Strapped on a pair of cross-country skis? Ice-skated? Roared down a hill on a toboggan? Now's your chance. Maintaining your workout program through the winter months—or starting an exercise regimen—will help keep your metabolism revved. Paying a trainer in advance will help get you started or keep you going. Why? No play, you still pay.

■ Be realistic about your goals. Aim to maintain, not gain, during the holidays. It's unrealistic to expect to lose weight during this period, and such a fantasy may set you up for disappointment. Make your goal not to lose a set number of pounds but to stick to your eating plan and work out as much as your holiday schedule allows.

■ Sample, rather than gorge, on holiday foods. After all, it's the first bite or two of cake, candy, or pie that tastes the best.

■ Get enough sleep. I don't mean to sound like your mother, but it's true that we often eat more when we're tired.

DANGER ZONE #32

TOOLS: 103, 104, 144, 202, 204

You're from a culture where food is equated with love.

In some cultures, to offer food is the ultimate expression of love—and to refuse it is the equivalent of an insult.

But consider this: We're raised to believe that if we refuse food, we're being rude. But if food is politely declined, then it's just as rude to insist that we accept it. Here's how to fend off Aunt Ida's pierogies—and her pushiness.

- If Aunt Ida always makes your favorite foods when you come to visit, ask her to make one dish that tends to be lower in fat and calories and that will help you stick to your program. She may love fussing in the kitchen, making this dish "especially for you."

- Or ask in advance what she plans to serve so that you can fit it into your program. Watch what you eat for the rest of the meal so you can enjoy that "just for you" dish.

- Before you visit, visualize your food-pushing relative as she puts a plate of your favorite dish in front of you and insists that you eat. How do you respond? What will you do if she won't take no for an answer?

- If you're invited to dinner, plead another appointment but say you'd love to drop by before dinner. Leave before the goodies are put on the table. Or say you'll stop by after dinner, when you suspect that the food is put away.

- Try Scarlett O'Hara's old trick: Eat something before you go so you're not overly hungry.

- Say you're not hungry now but that you'd love to take home a plate for later. Before you get home, toss it in the garbage.

- As you knock on the door, focus on this fact: You are an adult, and you get to decide what or whether you will eat. It's not unreasonable to say no to food you don't want, and you needn't be apologetic or embarrassed to say it.

DANGER ZONE #33 | TOOLS: 44, 53, 81, 92, 130, 152, 199

Ever since you stopped smoking, you can't stop eating.

An hour after your last cigarette, every pore in your body seemed to scream for chocolate. You answered their call—now you're 10 pounds heavier. Don't lose hope. Just stick to your eating plan and exercise regularly.

If you worry that extra "quit weight" puts your health at risk, relax: You'd have to gain from 100 to 150 pounds after quitting to make your health risks as high as when you smoked!

- Walk to keep from puffing—and eating. In one study, women who stopped smoking and walked 45 minutes a day gained less than 3 pounds.

- If you don't work out now, *start* now and set a smoking quit date for several months down the road. While everyone is different, many people find it extremely difficult to quit smoking at the same time they start an exercise program.

- Once you quit, brush your teeth after every meal. It will help break the powerful link between finishing a meal and lighting up.

- If you can't stop eating, keep your mouth busy with lollipops. (Sugarless, if you can.)

- Get fired up. Take inspiration from this ex-smoker's story, taken from *The No-Nag, No-Guilt, Do-It-Your-Own-Way Guide to Quitting Smoking* by Tom Ferguson, M.D.: "When I quit smoking, I gained 12 pounds. Determined to lose it, I drove to a supermarket 2 miles from home, marched up to the butcher counter, and had them grind me 12 pounds of hamburger. I left my car in the parking lot and carried it home. By the time I got home, I was exhausted. I was carrying that much extra weight around with me every day—no wonder I felt tired all the time! I gave most of the hamburger away to friends and neighbors, then started a running program the next day. I eventually shed those 12 pounds."

DANGER ZONE #34 | TOOLS: 40, 50, 62, 97, 142, 161, 210

Your colleagues bring doughnuts to work.

Or they have candy dishes on their desks and throw lots of birthday parties—with cake. The office is a breeding ground for Diet Danger Zones. With so many tempting choices in easy reach, it can be difficult to abstain. Here's how to withstand that 9-to-5 temptation.

- You're most vulnerable to this Diet Danger Zone if you're a meal skipper. Try to eat breakfast in the morning. You may be less likely to scarf a jelly doughnut at 10:30 A.M. And eat lunch so you won't wander over to colleagues who bear candy dishes.

- Take a healthy breakfast to work. Eat that when you'd normally reach for that jelly doughnut.

- If it's passing the snacks in the coffee or break room on your way to the fax machine or copier that tempts you, go the long way or take a different route.

- Take snacks to work and keep them in the office refrigerator or your desk drawer. Low-fat yogurt or sliced veggies are a better alternative to a stale doughnut anyway.

- At office birthday parties, mingle with your colleagues until the cake is cut. Then return to your desk.

- Carry sugarless gum. Pop a piece before you visit a colleague who keeps a candy dish on his desk.

- Sip from a bottle of water while others eat. It gives you something to do with your hands and reminds you of your weight-loss or weight-maintenance goals.

You're a chocolate addict.

According to a research study in the *Journal of the American Dietetic Association*, it's estimated that 40 percent of women crave chocolate, with a heightened desire for it before or during menstruation. Here's how to enjoy chocolate—just not too much of it.

- Indulge in premeasured doses. Chocolate is like plutonium: You need only a little to get the desired result. Keep five chocolate kisses on hand and, when you have a craving, allow yourself five. You'll consume just 125 calories.

- Don't think a small amount of chocolate can fully satisfy you? Try tool 56: Take a chocolate-appreciation break.

DANGER ZONE #36

TOOLS: 55, 56, 157, 186

You get pregnant and gain 15 pounds in the first trimester.

Weight gain in the first 3 months of pregnancy is often the hardest to lose because it's not baby weight—it's all yours. These tips assume that you've had the baby, you're not breastfeeding, and you're not pregnant again.

- To reduce the calories and increase the nutritional value of your meals, eat more vegetables and drink more water.

- Now that you're no longer indulging pregnancy-related cravings, replace the junk food in your pantry and cupboards with healthful foods.

- Choose your snacks with the goal of having them help you meet your nutritional goals. Low-fat yogurt and cheese contain calcium; fruits and vegetables are chock-full of healthy fiber; whole grain bread contains more nutrients than white.

- Once you have your child, use him as your "excuse" to exercise. Push him in a stroller through the park. Once he's old enough to hold up his head—and with your pediatrician's okay—strap him on the back of your bike and go. Talk about resistance training!

You hit menopause and gain 15 pounds overnight.

Once we hit perimenopause, metabolism, the body's internal calorie burner, can slow as much as 15 percent. And it's mainly because we let our muscles go soft. After 40, we tend to replace calorie-burning muscle with do-nothing fat. During perimenopause, we lose an average of ½ pound of muscle each year; during menopause, 1 pound a year. The less muscle we have, the fewer calories we burn. If you're 40 now, you could be down about 15 pounds of muscle—and burn from 600 to 750 fewer calories a day—by your 55th birthday!

While this is a frustrating situation, there are steps you can take to wrest back your waistline.

■ Accept the fact that it's harder to lose weight as you grow older. You will lose it but at a slower pace.

■ The research is very clear: Exercise is key. Perimenopausal or menopausal women who work out a lot do not gain as much weight as those who don't. So go to the gym but also go for walks, play tennis, swim, whatever. Become more active than you ever thought you would—or could!

■ Consider starting a weight-training program. Weight-training and other resistance exercises can help maintain and even increase muscle mass at any age. The more muscle mass you have, the more calories you use up, both while exercising and at rest.

■ To battle a flagging metabolism, eat smaller meals. Research out of Tufts University found that when older women eat small meals (250 and 500 calories), they burn fat as efficiently as younger women. But when they eat large meals (more than 1,000 calories), their metabolism's ability to burn fat is greatly impaired.

■ Don't give up. If nothing else, upping your activity level and eating fewer calories will stop you from *gaining* weight—and will eventually help you lose it.

DANGER ZONE #38

You stick to your diet Monday through Friday afternoon . . . and blow it over the weekend.

This is a common Diet Danger Zone, and it stems from the idea of "banking" your calories—starving during the week so you can cut loose, foodwise, over the weekend. This tactic rarely works, however. Here's what will.

- Get out of the house. Try hiking, biking, walking, or gardening. In bad weather, get to the gym or walk in the mall (if you can avoid the temptation of those jumbo cinnamon buns).

- Answer the following question: When it comes to weekend eating, how do fun and food collide? Perhaps the fun is meeting your friends at a pub, but the risk is in drinking 3 pints of lager and sharing plate after plate of mozzarella cheese sticks and Buffalo wings.

- Once you pinpoint the ground zero of food and fun, plan accordingly. In the example above, you might alternate each pint with a diet soda or plain water and keep the munchies on the other side of the table where you can't reach them.

- If you tend to wander in and out of the kitchen on the weekends, stock up on low-calorie finger foods such as baby carrots, cherry tomatoes, sliced cucumbers, and chopped-up fruit on Thursday night.

- If your hobby is trying new restaurants on the weekends, do something new. Food doesn't have to be the highlight of Saturday night. Take in a play or art exhibit with a friend, go bowling, go to a planetarium to see the midnight laser-light show.

You skip breakfast and lunch, then inhale the contents of the refrigerator at dinner.

One of the most damaging Diet Danger Zones is habitually fasting during the day and packing all your calories into one huge dinner. Skipping breakfast and lunch sends your body a message: "Uh-oh. Food supplies are scarce and unpredictable. I'd better conserve my energy and protect my fat stores." Which is exactly what you *don't* want it to do. Still, habits are hard to break, and it would be silly to tell you to eat breakfast if you're not really awake until noon. The tips below can help meal skippers get into the habit of eating during the day.

- If you're not a breakfast eater, it's okay not to start. (There's really no conclusive proof that eating breakfast benefits adults.) But it's not okay to starve all day. So eat lunch as well as a snack between lunch and dinner. You'll be less hungry come dinnertime.

- If you don't have time to consider what to have for lunch, opt for a turkey sandwich. Preferably a turkey sandwich on whole grain bread with mustard—hold the cheese, extra lettuce, onion, and tomato. This formulaic approach to lunch will help reduce impulse decisions so that you'll stay within your daily calorie allotment.

- Try to eat at least one-third your daily calories by the end of lunch. This will keep your energy levels high and your metabolism running efficiently.

- Make time for meals. If you're a breakfast skipper, get up 10 minutes earlier so you have time to make toast or grab a bowl of cereal. If you tend to forgo lunch, use the scheduling software on your computer to remind you to eat.

You have a diet "supervisor."

This is a friend (or parent or partner) who keeps track of everything you eat and finds it necessary to comment on your choices ("Should you be eating that?"). Even if they have your best interests at heart, these folks are walking Diet Danger Zones. Their comments can breed negative feelings about your eating plan, which will make you less likely to stick with it. Try these suggestions.

- Be honest without being rude. Say, "I'm sure you're saying what you're saying because you're trying to be supportive. But it would be more helpful to me if you could offer support by _____." Then tell them what you need from them or how they might be able to help you achieve your goals.

- In a quiet moment, think of a witty (yet not hurtful) comeback. You might say, "Hmm. Let me think about that. Yes, I should be eating this. I definitely should." Or "Amazing what science can accomplish these days. This plate of pasta is actually cottage cheese and melba toast."

- If they're friends or colleagues, rather than family, don't eat around them anymore. You don't need the aggravation. But if you enjoy their company, meet them for a game of Scrabble, a movie, or a brisk walk.

Part 4

MORE PATHS
TO SUCCESS

The Ultimate Weight-Loss
Weapon: A Pen

Here sat Jane, telling me she didn't understand why she'd gained 10 pounds after a year of successfully maintaining her weight loss.

"Have you scoured your food diary for clues?" I asked.

"No," Jane replied. "I don't need to keep a diary anymore. Believe me, my eating hasn't changed."

"Are you sure about that?" I asked.

Jane wasn't. So she went home and reluctantly wrote down what she'd eaten the day before. She then compared it with her last food-diary entry, recorded 6 months ago.

She was abashed at what she found.

Six months ago, breakfast was 1 ounce of bran flakes, 4 ounces of fat-free milk, and 1 cup of strawberries. Yesterday, it was a bran muffin and 4 ounces of orange juice.

Lunch used to be a cup of tomato soup and a turkey sandwich. Yesterday, she actually ate less: low-fat yogurt with fruit.

But dinner—that was a different story.

Six months ago, she'd opted for 6 ounces of steamed shrimp, 1 cup of broccoli, ⅔ cup of rice, a salad, and a glass of wine. Yesterday, she'd eaten Chinese—roast pork lo mein. What was the portion size? She hadn't a clue. (She'd ordered a "small.") No telling how many calories were in it either.

Her snacks? Their quality was about the same, but their quantity had risen greatly. Yesterday, she'd eaten three cookies during the day and had a noshfest at night—a handful of Cheerios, a box of raisins, some saltines, a peach, a slice of fat-free cheese . . .

Six months ago, she was consuming 1,550 calories a day. Now, she hadn't a clue.

The next day, Jane relaunched her food diary. She was relentless, recording everything from the cookie she'd eaten at 10:25 A.M. and the fingerful of frosting from a colleague's birthday cake at 3:45 P.M. to the 3 ounces of chicken, ½ cup of rice, and 1 cup of steamed veggies at 6:30 P.M.

Two weeks after she started her self-monitoring anew, she'd lost 2 pounds.

Such is the power of a food diary.

The Write Tool for Weight Control

If you've ever kept a journal, you know that it's a wonderful way to chronicle and make sense of the events in your life. Writing in your journal brings you closer to your true self. As such, it's a powerful tool for personal growth.

So is a food journal.

A food journal is much like a regular journal, except that the focus is on your eating. And if you're determined to lose weight, picking up that pen can increase your odds.

In clinical weight-loss programs, having people record what they eat is the best predictor of weight loss. It's also one of the best ways to maintain that loss. Research shows a strong relationship between keeping food records and meeting weight-loss goals.

Consider:

■ A group that kept detailed food diaries during a 15-week study lost 64 percent more weight than a group that didn't.

■ Out of 10 ways to alter eating habits, self-monitoring—that is, keeping a food diary—was the only one that allowed people to keep off their weight for up to 18 months.

■ In another study, 89 percent of the people who maintained their weight loss relied on food diaries.

■ Two studies showed that people who kept food diaries consistently lost more weight than those who kept track of their eating less than half the time. And only those who self-monitored consistently lost a significant amount of weight.

"I WILL" VERSUS "I SHOULD"

The point of this exercise is to give you an idea of what you're actually *willing* to do to lose weight or maintain your weight loss, rather than what you think you "should" do (which you most likely won't). Suppose the front page of the *New York Times* blares this headline: *Physicians Shocked: "Food Contains Twice the Calories We Thought!"* What would you do to lose weight or maintain your weight loss? Eat less? Give up certain foods? Exercise more? Just accept being fat?

When you consistently record what you eat, as you eat it, you become more aware of not only the food choices you make but also why and when you're most likely to make them. And with that awareness comes the potential for positive change.

"But I've Tried That Before!"

I'm betting many of you have already tried the food-diary thing and hated the whole experience. I can almost hear you: "It's boring. And I just don't have the time."

To which I reply: Do it anyway, because it works.

Or at least *try* to do it, even if you've tried before. It's possible that you haven't found the way to keep a food diary that's right for you and you alone.

That's right—there's more than one way to keep a food diary. There are probably dozens. So if counting calories is a crashing bore for you, don't. Find another way to record what you eat that makes sense to you, that you can live with. It doesn't matter how you "do" a food journal, as long as you do it and learn from it. Of course, the more you're willing to do to make your weight-control program a success, the better off you'll be.

That said, let me run down some of the benefits of keeping a food diary.

Diary Do's: Tips for Change

The first time you review your food diary, you may detect patterns or behaviors that are sabotaging your weight-control program. Here are the top 10 reasons you may be having problems and what to do about them.

10. *You're a nonstop nibbler.* Cart bushels of healthy, low-calorie produce into your house and slice, dice, and chop it up for ready consumption. It may reduce your urges to order takeout, to bring "binge foods" across your threshold, and to forage for food when you're tired or bored.

9. *You overeat between meals.* Limit yourself to just one kind of low-calorie food after a meal. It's easier to overeat when you have a variety of foods to choose from.

8. *You eat "because it's there."* Immediately call a support person and tattle on yourself. Saying out loud, "I've just ordered a triple-cheese pepperoni pizza, and it will be here in 30 minutes," may help you resist it when it arrives.

7. *You eat when you're angry or upset.* Open your diary and write a paragraph on who or what has upset you and what you would do if you were to let loose. "Binge" on words, as you might binge on a bag of chips or a box of cookies.

6. *You tend to overeat at mealtimes.* Divide the food on your plate in half. When you've eaten half, leave the table for a 10-minute break. Wash your face. Walk around the block. Slowly drink a tall

It can keep you honest. When it comes to weight loss, it's crucial to be unflinchingly honest about your eating. This can be difficult if, for you, eating is tangled up in shame or guilt. Many of my clients are so guilt-ridden about what they've eaten that they can't handle it and won't write it down. They ultimately go off their programs.

But as hard as it may be to confront your eating, keeping a food

glass of water. If you're in a restaurant or at a dinner party, excuse yourself and head to the powder room. This "downtime" can tame a raging appetite.

5. *You tend to "binge."* Cleanse your palate. If you're eating ice cream, switch to a sliced tomato. Cake? Try a slice of turkey. The radical change of taste can be like a slap in the face—a "thanks, I needed that" type of thing.

4. *You skip meals.* Stop that. Right now. You're setting yourself up for endless nibbling later. Or you may think it's okay to eat more—much more—because you've eaten so little up to now.

3. *You eat while you work or watch TV.* Designate one room in the house as your eating place—ideally, your dining room. (If you don't have a dining room, opt for the kitchen. And if you have a TV in your kitchen, pull the plug.)

2. *You snack between meals.* If you get hungry between meals, try breaking up your meals. For example, eat half your lunch at noon and the other half in the midafternoon. Or eat a large salad at dinnertime and the rest of your meal 2 or 3 hours later.

1. *You're an at-home eater.* Get out of the house. Sign up for a class, go to the library, play miniature golf, get your nails done. Avoid bookstores that proffer pastries.

diary allows you to take a clearer look at what, how much, and why you eat. There's incredible power in knowing that information.

It can keep you in control. Keeping a food diary takes the guesswork—and the guilt—out of eating. Say you eat a heavy lunch: 400 calories more than you'd planned. Recording what you ate and its calorie count immediately allows you to plan the rest of that day's eating. Knowing that you've got just 300 more calories to "spend," you'll be able to scale down your dinner and evening snacks.

It can help you formulate and meet goals. Once you get used to keeping your diary, you may want to set daily, weekly, or monthly eating or exercise goals. Each time you open your journal, you'll remember what you're striving for.

It serves as an early-warning system. Keeping a food diary can alert you to changes in your eating patterns before you see changes on the scale. So chances are good that you'll never have to experience the frustration of regaining lost pounds.

How to Keep a Food Diary

It's not rocket science, friends. Get a dime-store notebook and a pen. Then start tallying every last morsel of food that passes your lips.

If you've never kept a food diary, you may want to start with the traditional approach, in which you record the type and amount of food you eat for breakfast, lunch, dinner, and snacks. Total the calories for each meal, then for the entire day. (Don't forget to record the syrup on your waffle, the hard candies you had in a colleague's office, the nibbling you did as you prepared dinner.)

After that, you can include any other information you want. Some of my clients who keep traditional food diaries include:

- Where they ate

- What they were doing when they ate

- How fast they ate

- How they were feeling when they ate

- Whether or not they were actually hungry (and if they weren't, what other than hunger may have triggered their eating)

- How many grams of fat or carbohydrate they consumed

- Whether they met their dietary goals (for example, whether they consumed the number of fruits and vegetables or glasses of water they aim for each day)

"NET THERAPY": THE NEWEST WEIGHT-LOSS TOOL?

Behavioral therapy is the most effective treatment for obesity. But getting folks to behavioral-therapy programs isn't always easy.

What would happen if behavioral therapy came to the overweight rather than the other way around?

That's what researcher Deborah F. Tate, Ph.D., and her colleagues at Brown University School of Medicine in Providence, Rhode Island, wondered. So they studied 91 overweight men and women to determine whether a behavioral program, delivered over the Internet, would help folks lose more weight than weight-loss education alone.

These researchers, which included Rena R. Wing, Ph.D., cofounder of the National Weight-Loss Registry, broke their volunteers into two groups. One group got weight-loss education—access to a Web site loaded with links to information about diet, exercise, self-monitoring, and other resources.

The second group received behavioral therapy delivered via the Internet. This group kept food and exercise diaries and e-mailed them to a therapist each week. They also received individualized feedback from a behavioral therapist based on their weekly diary entries, a weekly weight-loss "lesson" via e-mail, and access to an online electronic bulletin board to find social support if they wanted it.

After 3 months, the interactive group was eating significantly fewer calories and expending significantly more calories in exercise. The interactive group had also lost an average of 8.8 pounds compared with the education group's 3.7-pound average.

There's no way to prove which component of the online therapy—the diaries, the individualized feedback, or both—produced the results. But the study seems to suggest that the Internet's ability to bring people together may be yet another tool in the battle against obesity.

Your journal should be small so that you can carry it with you everywhere. If it's too large to fit in your pocket or purse and you keep it at home, you may "forget" what you've eaten by the end of the day or not keep the diary at all.

LOATHE FOOD DIARIES? LOOK AT THESE

If you've kept a traditional food diary and hated it, I bring you tidings of great joy. Not one of these six alternatives requires you to crunch calories. Just make sure your diary is small, so you can tuck it into your pocket or purse and record at the table, in the restroom, anywhere.

The problem: You fall prey to occasional pig-outs.

The diary: The overeating food journal.

Try keeping a food diary in which you record only those times when you feel your eating got out of control. You might have 3 such times in a week or 10 in one day. Or you might run into trouble just on weekends. Just knowing your diary is with you may discourage you from impulsive overeating.

The problem: You're a TV muncher.

The diary: The hand-to-mouth food journal.

This diary can help you become aware of hand-to-mouth behavior (so named because it's the act of moving the hand to the mouth—not the food—that's important). Keep your diary near the remote. When the fact that you're eating beer nuts or cheese crunchies penetrates your consciousness, you can choose to continue eating them, opt for a lower-calorie snack, or choose not to eat at all.

The problem: You're a social eater.

The diary: The social-butterfly food diary.

If dining out is your Danger Zone, this diary asks that you record what you consume in a social setting in real time. So if you have three slices of garlic bread, you're already aware of it before you bite into the fourth.

The problem: You're a sneak eater.

The diary: The come-out-of-the-closet food journal.

Perhaps you eat like a bird when you're around others but overeat in private. Try keeping a diary of what you eat only when you're alone. Write, "I'm about to eat an entire box of glazed doughnuts." It's possible that simply admitting to what you're about to do makes doing it unnecessary.

The problem: You don't stop eating until you're in physical pain.

The diary: The fullness food journal.

For some, there's no such thing as being a "little" full. By the time they feel full, they're physically uncomfortable. If this sounds like you, try this diary.

In your diary, make three columns. Over each, write the headings: Comfortable, Too Full, and Stuffed. After you eat, make a check mark in the column that describes how you feel physically.

Underneath the check mark, list your physical symptoms. For example, if you choose the Stuffed column, you might write "tired," "nauseated," "have a stomachache," and so on. If you choose the Comfortably Full column, describe the physical sensations associated with fullness.

What does being comfortably full actually feel like? It's an absence of the physical symptoms we relate to eating—neither hunger nor being physically unable to move. If you don't know what that sensation feels like, here's how to find out. Eat half your meal. Then ask yourself the following questions. Record your answers in your diary.

- Do I have to loosen my belt?
- Do I feel lethargic?
- Could I have eaten less and not been hungry?

If you answered yes to these questions, you're probably overly full.

Now ask yourself, "Could I leave the table right now and not feel hungry?" If you answer yes, that's exactly how you want it!

The problem: You eat when you're sad, mad, anxious, or stressed.
The diary: The food-mood journal.

This diary weakens the powerful link between feelings and food because it helps you confront and analyze your emotional eating episodes.

In your notebook, make four columns: Food, Mood, Position, and How I Ate. When your emotions lead you to food (whether before, during, or after you eat), complete each column. Here are two sample entries.

• *Food:* Crunchy, salty, and fatty (chips). Then went to sweets (chocolate chip cookies). *Mood:* Angry. *Position:* Paced on the phone as I ate. *How I Ate:* Fast, with fingers, out of the box and bag. Didn't taste the food but was aware of the crunch of the chips. Anger seemed soothed with the soft cookies.

• *Food:* Comfort foods: melted cheese (in microwave), instant mashed potatoes, pudding, ice cream. *Mood:* Stressed. *Position:* Sitting/lying on living-room couch with TV on. *How I Ate:* Used no utensils; ate everything with fingers except for ice cream.

Playing Detective

If you've ever fantasized about being Nancy Drew or a Hardy Boy, you may come to enjoy keeping your food diary. Recording what you eat is only part one of the equation. Part two—the intriguing part—is using your diary to answer this question: *What's my motive for eating?*

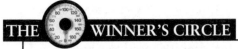

"I KNOW THAT EVERYTHING I PUT INTO MY MOUTH COUNTS"

Larry Hofrichter, of Highland Park, New Jersey, has a major Danger Zone. Faced with too many food choices, he loses control.

That's why the 54-year-old attorney avoids choices. "Left to my own devices, it's not a good result," he says wryly.

Instead, he sticks to more or less the same menu each day. And with this tool alone, he lost more than 75 pounds from his 5-foot 11-inch frame.

"Eating basically the same thing every day works well for me, and I don't get bored," says Hofrichter. "I now eat more often and more regularly—and the portions are large. For me, it's just a smarter way to eat."

Hofrichter's "smart menu" starts with cold cereal and milk for breakfast, a meal he rarely ate before his weight loss. Lunch is a large salad topped with grilled chicken. Dinner? Another sizable portion of greens and a frozen dinner. If he gets hungry at night, he has a fruit plate.

On Friday nights, Hofrichter, who is Jewish, celebrates the Sabbath with challah bread, a large piece of grilled or broiled salmon, and lots of steamed carrots, broccoli, mushrooms, and onions, together with the ever-present large salad.

Using tools has helped him become aware of—and thereby take control of—his food choices. "It's not constant nitpicking. It's constant awareness," he says. "I know that everything I put into my mouth counts."

Before he began using tools, "there were virtually no limits to what or when I would eat," says Hofrichter. "I ate huge amounts irregularly and all day on the weekends."

As you'll probably discover, we often don't have a motive. Much of the time, we eat on autopilot.

Think of the times you've munched from a jumbo bag of chips. Were you aware of how many you ate? Right. Did you taste each chip? Not likely. But once you launch a food diary, you'll be exquisitely aware of everything you put into your mouth.

Keeping food records is a critical tool for him, he says, because it forces him to take responsibility for every nibble and nosh. It's important because while he usually sticks to his maintenance plan pretty well, he says, "There are times when I'm sitting in front of the TV in the evening, having pretzels, and I know I'm having too many."

Moreover, Hofrichter's good intentions are frequently challenged by restaurant lunches and other business-related events. Keeping a running tab of his food intake helps rein him in. "I've found that when I focus on my food records, I focus on the strategies that help me control my eating," he says.

Making time for regular physical activity is a bit more challenging. "I ride a stationary bike and lift weights sporadically," he says. "I'm trying to get back into the exercise habit."

For now, his primary move tool is "nickel-and-dime" activity—making more trips to the attic, taking the stairs instead of elevators and escalators, walking to the water cooler, and taking documents to the photocopier one at a time so that he makes more trips.

"I've ordered a pedometer, though, so I can aim for taking a certain number of steps each day," he says.

Other favorite tools are rules for dealing with favorite foods, eating only in the dining room or at the kitchen table, avoiding tasteless but high- (or low-) calorie foods, getting half or more of his calories from vegetables, varying food records and other assessment tools, telling a friend (support from spouse), and having fixed (acceptable) meals at favorite restaurants.

I believe everyone should use their food diary every day, but to detect your eating pattern and behavior, you'll need to keep it for at least 3 days. But ideally, you'll want to record for at least 2 full weeks, so you can see if your weekday eating pattern differs from your weekend one.

So, amateur sleuth, here's what to look for as you pore over your diary entries.

- How many times a day did you eat?

- How many times did you simply pop something into your mouth because it was there?

- How many meals did you have? How many snacks? Compare the two.

- Is there a calorie difference between snacks and meals? How much of a difference?

- Do you eat differently during the week than on weekends? How?

- Is your eating pattern stable or erratic? In other words, do you eat pretty much the same thing, at the same time, day after day, or does your pattern vary wildly depending on your schedule or mood?

Some of my clients have lost weight after keeping their diary for less than a week. There's no magic here. They simply became conscious of when, where, and how much they ate and were able to put on the brakes.

What's Up with Jane's Diet?

At the beginning of this chapter, you met Jane. I thought it would be helpful to critique her diary entries so you can get an idea of how to read your own.

When I analyze a food record, I look at three things: eating pattern (how many times a day a person eats), food choice, and volume. Let's see how Jane's food record of 6 months ago stacks up against her recent one.

Eating pattern. While Jane is still eating three meals a day, she's snacking more.

Food choice. Jane appears to be eating more of what I call "I Don't Know" foods than she was 6 months ago. "I Don't Know" foods are those that are impossible to calculate calorie-wise. Case in point: her breakfast bran muffin. How big was it? Three ounces or one of those monster muffins that are as big as your fist? Did it pack 300 calories or 800? How many calories were in her pint of roast pork lo mein? There's no way to tell—and that's a problem.

To get back on track, Jane may want to stick to simple foods made with basic ingredients, like cereal and milk and fruits and vegetables. If she craves Chinese, she can opt for ½ cup of steamed white or brown rice and a steamed entrée rather than a selection smothered in an "I Don't Know" sauce.

Volume. Jane isn't eating more than she was a year ago. In fact, at lunch, she's eating significantly less. But take a look at her after-dinner snacks. She's nibbling a lot, which indicates that she's dissatisfied with her choices, her portion sizes, or both.

Or it could be that she's eating more at night because she's not eating enough during the day. Jane would do better to eat a heartier lunch. Going back to eating her soup and sandwich combo may help her avoid night eating, which could eventually get out of control.

The Final Frontier:
Weight-Loss Maintenance

My client Lisa is a poster child for weight maintenance.

Several years ago, the 59-year-old child psychologist came to me for help in losing weight. She succeeded, ultimately shedding 77 pounds. More impressive, she kept them off for more than a year.

Lisa appeared to be the perfect fitness-magazine success story. Then her life began to change. Unhappily, so did her weight.

Distracted by her hectic life, Lisa found it harder and harder to meet with me for her weekly appointments and to make her group sessions. She was also confronting a stressful job situation, which triggered non-stop nibbling. Within 5 months, she regained 17 pounds and hovered at that weight for another few years.

Then she got uterine cancer, which completely turned her life inside out. Frightened and depressed, Lisa tried to soothe her emotional pain with food. Her cancer treatments also caused her to gain weight.

Ultimately, Lisa recovered. But her health crisis ended with her having regained all 77 pounds . . . plus 10 more, which was a health crisis in itself.

As a cancer survivor, Lisa knew it was risky for her to stay fat. Somehow, she found the courage to make it back to my office.

Lisa also had something else going for her: prior experience with maintenance. After all, she'd once kept most of her lost pounds lost for more than a year. So she knew what maintenance entailed for her, personally, now to maintain her weight loss for good.

Since that day, Lisa has lost 89 pounds and has kept them off for 2 years. She's not at her ideal goal—a size-14 dress—but she is at a healthy weight.

"For me, the most important part of maintenance is knowing that I

HE CRAVES, SHE CRAVES

If you're a woman, you may have wondered why you never see your guy huddled on the couch spooning cookie-dough ice cream from the container when he's feeling blue. A French study of over 1,000 men and women of normal weight may provide a clue.

The study linked food cravings to mood states. That's no surprise. But get this: When it comes to the *moods* that trigger their cravings, men and women are just about opposites.

The study found that while both men and women crave particular foods, women are twice as likely as men to report cravings (28 percent of women versus 13 percent of men).

What's more, women report having the strongest cravings when they're sad. Men, on the other hand, said their cravings were most powerful when they were happy.

And perhaps to no one's surprise, the study also found that cravers—especially female cravers—reported feeling more concerned about their weight than noncravers.

can survive the lapses, which are no longer failures to me but a part of life," she says. "I keep track better than I ever did. When I resort to my old ways, I take action quickly. And I'm confident now that as long as I stay aware, I can get back—and stay—on track."

Maintenance: A State of Mind

I tell this story because you need to understand that moving from weight loss to weight-loss maintenance isn't easy. Most people know how to lose and gain. Few know how to maintain.

Some people in maintenance continue to "diet," restricting their food intake until they hallucinate cheeseburgers and revert to their old ways. Others, like Lisa, go through life changes that cause them to fall off the wagon, so to speak. When life changes, priorities can change, too. And healthy eating and regular exercise can suddenly take a backseat without your being aware of it.

I'm sure this sounds discouraging. But I'd be doing you a disservice if I didn't warn you of the pitfalls of weight maintenance.

But there *is* good news. More people succeed at maintenance than researchers previously thought, and many keep off the weight longer than they used to.

We know what successful weight maintainers *do*, thanks to the folks enrolled in the National Weight Control Registry (NWCR). (For more on the NWCR, see "Don't Swallow These Weight-Loss Myths" on page

THE WINNER'S CIRCLE

"I DON'T HAVE TO BE A SAINT"

Tracey Dye regards her weight loss as part of a larger life plan to "get healthier and get grounded." In fact, she's finding that as she sheds her extra pounds, she's also shedding some pretty heavy emotional baggage.

"I've been struggling with weight since I was a child," says Dye, 33, a graduate student in anthropology and teacher of English as a second language. "Through therapy, I continue to recognize how susceptible I am to undermining myself."

Yet thanks to Cathy's tools and an unwavering commitment to change old habits, Dye says she's never felt better. While she doesn't have a clue how many pounds she's lost—she doesn't use scales—Dye uses other things to gauge success: an increase in muscle tone, pants and skirts that hang on her, and the emergence of knees, wrists, and cheekbones.

One of the tools she depends on most is the food diary. She records everything she eats, even if it's a Pop-Tart or two for dinner. A food record, she says, helps her stay grounded. "I'm aware of those instances—which are pretty rare—when I don't pay attention to what I'm eating. My food diary allows me to dissect why I didn't pay attention."

Exercise is another critical tool for Dye, a committed walker. As

225.) They exercise a lot. They follow a low-fat diet. They use food diaries.

But how do they manage to do what they have to do, day after day, year after year?

There are clues that offer us hope—and a path.

There's a saying, well-known by the folks in Alcoholics Anonymous, that to me gets at the essence of maintenance: "Progress, not perfection."

People who manage to lose weight and maintain that loss have come to terms with the fact that while dieting has an end, maintenance

---

her schedule changes, she works hard to squeeze walks into her varied routine.

To keep a stash of healthy snacks and meals on hand, Dye spends Sundays cutting up veggies and preparing healthy salads that she can grab for lunch. "Home is not an issue," she says. "When it comes to food choices, I feel more unsafe outside my home than inside it."

For that reason, Dye uses a variety of tools to prepare for invitations to friends' homes or restaurants. She'll bring a healthy chicken dish to a chum's dinner party, for instance, and drink lots of water during the evening so she is not tempted by high-calorie treats or wines or liquors that could melt her resolve.

If a pal invites her to a bar for drinks, she'll offer an alternative date. "I try not to get in situations where people say, "Oh, come on and eat," Dye explains.

If she must enter a favorite deli, Dye will buy bottled water and drink that to avoid fattening temptations.

Yet part of Dye's plan is to include ice cream and other treats she adores. "I don't have to be a saint," she says. "I don't have to do it right all the time."

doesn't. They know maintenance is a one-day-at-a-time proposition. They also know that slips happen, and that when they do, their ultimate success depends on responding quickly and thoughtfully.

This knowledge comes with experience. Successful maintainers have lived through every season, every holiday, any number of food-oriented social events. They've analyzed their eating patterns and behavior in these situations, learned what works for them and what doesn't, and learned to use tools to avoid their Diet Danger Zones. They don't get cocky, and they self-monitor to ensure that they're staying on the straight and narrow. All of these behaviors help them respond constructively to lapses.

So while we can't define maintenance, we can describe it. In maintenance, you're not dieting unless you're doing it to get back on track. You're rarely nervous about "being good" when you go out to dinner because you have a lot of dining experience under your belt (which has gone down a size or two, thank you). You don't live in fear of stepping on the scale because you know whether you're in control of your eating—or out of control.

So what *are* you doing? Read on.

Maintainer, Evaluate Thyself

By now, you may suspect that maintenance is about more than a number on a scale. It's a state of mind, reinforced with concrete strategies to prevent or respond to slips.

It's also about the ability to *evaluate*—to monitor the state of your maintenance, if you will. Successful maintainers don't leave that success to chance. They're constantly monitoring their eating and exercise patterns and staying alert for potential pitfalls—from lifestyle changes to stress or negative thinking—that might sabotage their efforts.

Evaluation is the name of the maintenance game, so don't neglect it. Here's my short list of "do's" for long-term weight-maintenance success.

Do track your progress. Maintenance is about achieving a higher level of consciousness about food, physical activity, and your Diet Danger Zones. The best way to do this is to continually evaluate where

CULTIVATING "WINNER'S MIND"

Keeping lost pounds lost doesn't just "happen." Consider the importance of cultivating the qualities below.

1. Foresight. You're able to plan ahead to keep your program on track. You can also see potential threats to your program *before* they become a problem.

2. Resilience. You're able to get up and dust yourself off when you have a lapse or even a relapse.

3. Self-esteem. You're able to see that you're a worthy person who deserves to succeed, and you're able to ask for help when you need it. Also, you can see what you're doing *right*, rather than merely focusing on your mistakes.

Using the space below, list other qualities that you feel could increase your odds of successful maintenance. (More examples: honesty, the ability to calm yourself under stress, the ability to learn from lapses.) Why are they important? How might they help?

_____

_____

_____

_____

_____

_____

you are and where you need to be. So assess your progress daily, weekly, or at least monthly or quarterly, depending on the evaluation tools you choose.

The diary is the supreme evaluation tool. (See page 208 for more information on starting and keeping a diary.) One client of mine starts to record her food intake any time she gains 5 pounds. If she gains 10, she e-mails her food records to me.

Other evaluation parameters include:

Your "numbers." Are your blood cholesterol, blood pressure, and blood sugar dropping? Staying steady? Spiking crazily up and down? Why? Has your dosage of medication changed? Have you been able to go off medication completely?

Your fitness level. How much weight can you lift during your resistance-training workouts? How many times can you lift it? How long and how hard can you walk? Is your percentage of body fat decreasing? Are your strength and endurance increasing?

Your goals. Are you regularly making new short-term goals and revising long-term goals? Are your goals realistic and achievable, and are you coming closer to achieving them?

Do evaluate your tools. Life changes. We move; fall in and out of love; switch jobs or retire; get sick; have children or watch those children leave the nest. And as our lives change, so must our weight-maintenance tactics.

To make tools work for you as effectively as possible, take an active role in choosing and using them—and discarding them, if necessary, when they no longer work. Some questions to ask yourself: Do my tools still work as well as they did when I first started using them, or have they stopped working? Has my life changed in any way, and do I need new tools to accommodate those changes and head off potential Diet Danger Zones?

For example, if you move from a workplace that has a cafeteria that offers fresh, healthy fare to one that offers vending-machine fare, you'll need to find tools that will help you avoid this potential Danger Zone. Or if you've established a running program but suddenly blow out your knee, you'll need to find tools that help you identify and stick to an alternative workout.

Do evaluate the changes you're willing to live with. To successfully transition from weight loss to weight maintenance, we must integrate what worked for us in our weight-loss phase into real life—stressful jobs, demanding families, endless obligations, and all. This means deciding which eating and exercise changes we can live with permanently and which we can't.

For example, you may be able to live with pouring fat-free milk into

The Top 10 Tenets of Maintenance Success

10. Remember how far you've come and why.

9. Evaluate your tools regularly.

8. Road test new tools often.

7. When life changes, adjust your tools. Seek out tools that can help you adapt to your changing circumstances.

6. Continue to devise new goals. You'll stay motivated and on your toes.

5. Remember that there's no such thing as cheating. There's just eating.

4. Remember that there are no "bad" days, just normal, occasional occurrences.

3. Eat plenty of vegetables. Then eat more.

2. Practice portion control.

1. Move as much as you can. Then move more.

your coffee rather than half-and-half and ordering steamed vegetables instead of french fries when you dine out. But if you aren't willing to give up your favorite gourmet ice cream, don't even try. However, you will need to decide if you can live with having one portion of the good stuff rather than a whole pint, the way you used to.

You also have to decide whether you can live with the tools you've chosen. It sounds obvious, but don't choose tools you think you "should" be using. Tools work only if you're willing to use them.

Each night before you go to bed, ask yourself if the tools you used today to maintain your weight are tools you could use for the rest of your life. If the answer is yes, then ask yourself if the tools helped you stay on course. If the answer is still yes, you'll know you're on the right

"IT'S DEFINITELY 'ENGAGE BRAIN BEFORE OPENING MOUTH'"

Since Dori Binn used her first tool almost 5 years ago, she's lost 137 pounds.

More important, she's kept them off.

The 43-year-old nuclear medicine technologist, who began working with Cathy in June 1997, has maintained her weight since October 1998. She credits tools for her success. "They're little tricks that happen to work really well—and they're simple to use."

One tool that works for Binn is to avoid starches such as bread, rice, and pasta. Another? Keeping food records, which she sometimes e-mails to Cathy for feedback.

She also drinks 5 to 7 liters of water a day. "I've learned that sometimes when you feel hungry, you're really thirsty," says Binn. "So before I eat, I'll often drink 32 ounces of a noncaloric liquid. Then, if I'm still hungry, I'll eat.

"It's definitely 'engage brain before opening mouth.'"

The fact that tools make you more aware of how and what you eat—and, often, *why* you're eating—is the primary reason they work so well, says Binn.

"Once you can connect your desire to eat with what's going on at that moment, it becomes easier to make a choice not to eat," she says. "And yet, I know that if there was anything I really, truly wanted to eat, I could have it. It's just a matter of 'Is eating it worth the payback?' Usually, it isn't."

Binn also uses move tools to keep herself active—a critical part of the weight-loss and weight-maintenance equation.

"I bike or walk for 30 minutes a day, every day, and lift weights 6 days a week," she says. She has also found ways to move more in her daily life.

As a bonus, as her weight has gone down, so have her cholesterol, blood sugar, and blood pressure.

Tools have helped show Binn that "weight maintenance is incredibly doable. People tend to see losing weight as climbing this huge mountain—'There's no way I can do this!' But they can. And tools can help."

DON'T SWALLOW THESE WEIGHT-LOSS MYTHS

Here's another lesson we can learn from the folks enrolled in the National Weight Control Registry (NWCR): Much of what we think is gospel about weight loss isn't. Consider these three myths.

Myth 1: If you were fat as a kid, it's impossible to lose weight as an adult. Not so fast. Two-thirds of NWCR enrollees were overweight as children, and 60 percent report a family history of obesity.

Myth 2: It's virtually impossible to lose weight after 40. It may be harder, but it's not impossible. The average NWCR participant is 45. Many are substantially older.

Myth 3: Only people who have a small amount of weight to lose can keep the weight off. Pish! The average NWCR enrollee has lost about 60 pounds and kept if off for 5 years!

path to building a new, healthier lifestyle. If the answer is no, find other tools you *can* live with.

Do make exercise a core part of your maintenance program. More than 80 percent of NWCR enrollees succeeded in maintaining their weight loss after they increased their physical activity. Men burned more than 3,500 calories a week exercising, while women burned almost 2,700 a week. Check out the Move Tools chapter (page 125) for inspiration.

Maintenance Don'ts

You worked hard to lose weight. Now you have to work hard to keep it off (although NWCR participants report that it gets easier over time). Just as you'll want to follow the principles above, you'll want to avoid the missteps below.

Don't ignore red flags. This is harder to do than it seems. Sometimes, people in maintenance can get a bit cavalier. But taking their healthy weight for granted is a luxury people in maintenance can't afford.

If you always gain 2 or 3 pounds the week before your period, fine.

But if you gained 5 or 6 pounds this month, heads up. Consider whether you hit the chocolate or Chinese food a bit more than normal or if you've gone from jogging four times a week to once.

Don't allow a lapse to lead to collapse. Everyone in maintenance lapses. But successful maintainers don't allow their lapses to become re-lapses (a string of lapses in a row) or collapse (a total derailment of their program).

When you have a lapse, get up, dust off, and repair the damage. Your repairs might include picking up your food diary if you've let it go, getting extra support from friends, or attending groups such as Weight Watchers or TOPS.

Or experiment with new tools. After a lapse, skim the tools in this book, pick one you've never tried, and try it. Taking an active step to get back on track, even if it doesn't work, will make you feel more in control.

Don't take an all-or-nothing view of maintenance. All-or-nothing thinking, in which you view foods as good or bad and your efforts to maintain your weight as perfect or a failure, can be the ruin of your program. This is faulty thinking, punctuated by "I should have," "If only I'd," and "I must."

Be on the lookout for episodes of black-or-white thinking and be ready with a response if you do succumb. One way to deal with it is to "talk it off." Counter every negative thought with a more positive one. So if you splurge one day out of seven, don't say, "I blew it! I'm off my program. I might as well give up." Rather, talk to yourself gently: "I overate today, but I forgive myself. It's only one hour, one evening, one day. If I stop now, I can move forward."

At the end of the day, diets are temporary, but maintenance is forever. So forgive yourself for yesterday. Do your best today. And if you have a slip, straighten your shoulders, hold your head high, and steal a line from the indomitable Southern belle Scarlett O'Hara:

"Tomorrow is another day."

Part 5

THE *OUTWIT YOUR WEIGHT* RECIPE TOOL KIT

Quick and Healthy Recipes for the 10 Most Treacherous Danger Zones

Whatever your Diet Danger Zones, one thing's for sure: You always have to eat. Another truism: More often than not, food prepared at home is lower in fat and calories than take-out or restaurant meals, if you learn to cook light and lean.

Still, if your definition of home cooking means skinless chicken breast and cottage cheese night after night, you'll soon run screaming to the nearest Domino's. You'll also be dissatisfied if you can't cook what you crave, be it crispy chips, savory pizza, luscious desserts, or stick-to-the-ribs meals like Mom used to make.

The solution? Using recipes as tools to help keep your Diet Danger Zones from sabotaging your program. Following, you'll find 10 of the most common Danger Zones, along with recipes that may make them easier for you to whip.

For example, if your biggest Danger Zone is chocolate, turn to the sumptuous chocolate recipes. If you're a weekend eater, check out the delicious meals you often crave on Friday and Saturday nights and Sunday morning, from steak sandwiches to French toast. If you tend to overeat during the winter months, try your hand at the hearty dishes made with slimmed-down ingredients. No matter what your Danger Zone, you're bound to find a recipe that will satisfy a craving in a healthy manner.

Of course, use common sense. You can't eat three servings of chocolate cake or five slices of pizza without gaining weight, even if they're prepared with lower-fat ingredients. Freeze leftovers in single-serving portions—or, if you prefer, simply throw them away.

Happy (and healthy) cooking!

TOP 14 PANTRY ESSENTIALS

Keep your cupboard, fridge, and freezer stocked with these foods and you'll always have the makings of a delicious, healthful dinner on hand. And don't forget *fresh* staples, such as lemons, limes, ginger, and garlic—seasoning foods that you can use to make any meal special.

1. Canned beans (all kinds: black, white, pink, pinto, kidney, lima, fat-free refried) for pureeing and using as spreads, tossing into salads, and making vegetarian chili. Beans add protein and fiber to any dish, and they are ready to use. (Rinse well to remove some of the excess sodium.) Try mashing and mixing them with brown rice and seasonings for homemade veggie burgers.

2. Broths (fat-free, reduced-sodium beef and chicken; vegetable; tomato) for sautéing and cooking with rice and grains, as well as for creating simple soups

3. Canned fish (salmon, smoked oysters, tuna) for sandwiches, salads, and pasta

4. Dried foods (fruits, tomatoes, mushrooms) to add to grain or rice pilafs

5. Whole grains (couscous, oatmeal, quick-cooking barley, bulgur) and rice (pilaf mixes, brown, white, jasmine, basmati, Texmati). Add a few seasonings for a side dish or layer them with meats and vegetables in a baking dish.

6. Nuts (almonds, hazelnuts, walnuts) to add to pilafs and to top vegetables such as green beans. (Refrigerate or freeze nuts once opened.) Chop finely and add to bread crumbs as a coating for fish or chicken. Toss into salads or stir into cooked rice for extra protein. (Don't get carried away—nuts are high in calories.)

7. Oils and vinegars (olive, canola, corn oils; white, cider, red and white balsamic, and fruit-flavored vinegars, such as raspberry) for cooking and salad dressing

8. Whole wheat pasta (assorted shapes and sizes, including small pastas for soups). Nothing can beat it for a quick and filling dinner.

9. Seasonings and condiments (assorted dried herbs and spices, ethnic seasoning mixes, mustard, chutneys) to add exotic flavor to simple foods such as rice and cheese dishes, casseroles, and stews

10. Tomato products (canned tomatoes, sauces, purees, pastes) for sauces, pizza toppings, soups, and stews. Stir into rice or other grains. Or just heat and serve stewed tomatoes over pasta. They're preseasoned and need no embellishment.

11. Marinated artichoke hearts. They add pizzazz to everything from appetizers to pizzas. Use the marinade to flavor rice and pasta salads, to sauté vegetables, or to season meat, fish, or vegetables for grilling.

12. Sliced olives and jalapeños. Stir into chili, pack into burritos, toss into pasta sauces. They add lots of flavor and need no prep.

13. Spice blends. Some favorites to try: fines herbes (a mixture of tarragon, chervil, and savory), lemon pepper (does the job of salt and pepper, with an extra tangy taste), and Cajun spices.

14. Evaporated fat-free milk. An instant substitute for heavy cream in soups, casseroles, sauces—with zero fat.

You're tired.

What you need: 15-minute meals

This Danger Zone refers to "fatigue eating," or nibbling in a misguided attempt to keep your eyes open. But it's also true that when you're drop-dead exhausted, it's easier to opt for a fat-laden take-out or restaurant meal. Not anymore. The recipes below won't take any longer to prepare than waiting in line at the typical fast-food drive-thru window—and they're healthier.

COMMONSENSE STRATEGY: Make the following meals on a lazy Sunday afternoon and freeze them in single-serving or family-size portions. Then, when after-work exhaustion hits, you have yourself a healthy, microwaveable meal. And more time to rest.

Peanut Noodles with Chicken and Watercress

Try this easy dish that requires virtually no cooking.

- 2 tablespoons light soy sauce
- 2 tablespoons mirin (see note)
- 2 tablespoons lime juice
- 1½ tablespoons dark brown sugar
- ⅓ cup creamy peanut butter
- ¼ teaspoon red-pepper flakes (optional)
- 8 ounces spaghetti
- 1 red bell pepper, thinly sliced
- 1 yellow bell pepper, thinly sliced
- 2 cups coarsely chopped watercress
- 1 pound smoked chicken breast, sliced or shredded

1. In a small bowl, mix the soy sauce, mirin, lime juice, and brown sugar. Stir in the peanut butter and red-pepper flakes (if using).

2. Cook the spaghetti according to package directions. Drain and transfer to a large bowl. Add the peanut sauce and toss well. Add the pepper slices and watercress. Mix well. Serve topped with the chicken.

Makes 6 servings

Per serving: 329 calories, 9 g fat, 40 mg cholesterol, 1 g fiber, 848 mg sodium

Note: Mirin is a sweet, golden, low-alcohol wine made from rice. Essential in Japanese cooking, this ingredient adds sweetness and flavor to many dishes. It is available in all Japanese markets and in the ethnic aisle of most supermarkets.

Garlicky Shrimp in Mustard Sauce

Here's a perfect shrimp solution for a midweek dinner.

1   tablespoon lemon juice

1   tablespoon Dijon mustard

4   teaspoons Worcestershire sauce

1   tablespoon olive oil

1½ pounds large shrimp, peeled and deveined

   Salt

2   teaspoons finely chopped garlic

1   teaspoon chopped parsley

1   teaspoon chopped fresh oregano

   Freshly ground black pepper

1. In a small bowl, mix the lemon juice, mustard, and Worcestershire.

2. Put the oil in a large skillet over high heat. Add the shrimp, season lightly with salt, and cook, stirring frequently, for 3 to 4 minutes, or until just cooked through. Reduce the heat to very low, stir in the garlic, and cook, stirring, for about 30 seconds.

3. Remove the skillet from the heat, add the sauce, and stir to coat the shrimp. Sprinkle with the parsley, oregano, and pepper.

Makes 6 servings

Per serving: 77 calories, 3 g fat, 72 mg cholesterol, 0 g fiber, 230 mg sodium

Poached Salmon with Toasted Bread Crumbs and Basil

High in heart-friendly omega-3 fatty acids, salmon is delicious and readily available.

- 1 **thin lemon slice**
- 1 **bay leaf**
- 2 **teaspoons olive oil**
- ¼ **cup dried bread crumbs**
- 1 **tablespoon chopped pine nuts or other nuts**
- 1 **clove garlic, finely chopped**
- 2 **tablespoons grated Parmesan cheese**
- 1 **tablespoon drained, chopped sun-dried tomatoes**
  Salt
  Freshly ground black pepper
- 2 **tablespoons chopped fresh basil**
- 4 **salmon fillets, ½" thick and 4 ounces each, with skin**

1. Put 4 cups of hot water and the lemon slice and bay leaf in a large skillet. Bring to a simmer over low heat.

2. Warm the oil in a small skillet over low heat. Stir in the bread crumbs and nuts and cook, stirring, for 2 minutes, or until lightly toasted. Add the garlic and cook, stirring, for 1 minute, or until the garlic is fragrant.

3. Turn off the heat and stir in the cheese and tomatoes. Season with the salt and pepper, then stir in the basil.

4. Place the fillets, skin side up, in the simmering water, adding more hot water if needed to just cover. Cook for 10 minutes, or until just cooked through. Transfer to a platter. Remove and discard the skin and bay leaf.

5. Turn the fillets over and spoon the bread crumb mixture on top.

Makes 4 servings

Per serving: 263 calories, 12 g fat, 65 mg cholesterol, 0 g fiber, 134 mg sodium

Homemade Pizza in a Flash

When you're beat and the kids are clamoring for pizza, don't do the takeout thing. Instead, make this quick and easy pie. Use any vegetables you like, such as red bell pepper slices, chopped artichoke hearts, and small broccoli florets.

1   frozen whole wheat pizza crust (1 pound), defrosted

1   cup fat-free pizza sauce

2   cups fresh vegetables

4   ounces soy mozzarella-style cheese or low-fat mozzarella cheese, shredded

1. Preheat the oven to 400°F.

2. Place the crust on a pizza pan. Spoon the sauce evenly over the crust. Top with the vegetables and sprinkle with the mozzarella cheese.

3. Bake for 10 to 15 minutes, or until the cheese is melted and the crust is lightly browned.

Makes 4 servings

Per serving: 325 calories, 9 g fat, 0 mg cholesterol, 4 g fiber, 797 mg sodium

Beefy Tortilla Stack

If you can't stomach jalapeño peppers, use black olives instead.
Serve with a tossed salad.

6	ounces cooked roast beef, cut into bite-size pieces
¼	teaspoon ground cumin
1	jar (16 ounces) garden-style salsa
6	whole wheat or corn tortillas (6" diameter)
6	tablespoons fat-free sour cream
1	can (15½ ounces) low-sodium black beans, rinsed and drained
½	cup sliced canned jalapeño peppers
2	tablespoons chopped fresh cilantro
1	cup shredded low-fat Monterey Jack cheese

1. Preheat the oven to 350°F. In a small bowl, toss together the beef and cumin.

2. Spread 2 tablespoons of the salsa in a 1½-quart round baking dish. Top with 1 tortilla and ⅙ of *each*: sour cream, beans, beef, peppers, cilantro, and cheese. Repeat layering (start each layer with salsa and end with cheese) until all ingredients are used. After adding each tortilla, press down slightly on stack to keep it level.

3. Bake for 15 to 20 minutes, or until the cheese is melted and the salsa is bubbling.

Makes 4 servings

Per serving: 415 calories, 15 g fat, 66 mg cholesterol, 11 g fiber, 27 mg sodium

Pork Chops with Mexican Peanut Sauce

A small amount of peanut butter lends a wonderful flavor and velvety texture to this sauce. If you like, garnish with fat-free sour cream and scallions.

4	lean, boneless pork chops, about 4 ounces each
3	teaspoons chili powder
1	can (8 ounces) no-salt-added tomato sauce
½–1	canned chipotle chile, seeded and chopped (see note)
2	tablespoons peanut butter
1	scallion, cut into 1" pieces
½	teaspoon instant coffee
½	teaspoon ground cinnamon

1. Sprinkle the pork on both sides with 2 teaspoons of the chili powder. Coat a skillet with cooking spray and place over medium heat until hot. Add the pork and cook for 5 minutes. Turn and cook for 5 minutes, or until the juices run clear. (The internal temperature should be 160°F.)

2. In a blender, combine the tomato sauce, chipotle, peanut butter, scallion, coffee, cinnamon, and the remaining 1 teaspoon chili powder. Blend until smooth. Transfer to a small saucepan and simmer for 4 minutes. Serve with the pork.

Makes 4 servings

Per serving: 257 calories, 13 g fat, 68 mg cholesterol, 2 g fiber, 200 mg sodium

Note: You can find chipotle chiles in small cans in the Mexican section of your supermarket. These chiles are actually smoked, dried jalapeño chile peppers cooked in a spicy tomato sauce called adobo. Remove the seeds, which contain most of the heat.

This recipe was created by Paul Piccuito.

Black Bean Burritos

Ingredients for this supper will have you sailing through the express line. Round the meal out with your favorite steamed or raw vegetables.

> 8   flour tortillas (6" diameter)
>
> 1   jar (12 ounces) fat-free black bean dip
>
> 1   cup shredded Monterey Jack cheese
>
> 1   package (10 ounces) prewashed shredded lettuce
>
> 1   small jar (10 ounces) salsa

1. Preheat the oven to 400°F.

2. Wrap the tortillas in a paper towel and microwave on high power for 30 seconds to soften.

3. Place 2 tablespoons of the bean dip, 2 tablespoons of the cheese, and a sprinkling of the lettuce in a line down the center of each tortilla. Roll up and place on a foil-lined tray. Place 1 tablespoon of the salsa over each roll.

4. Bake for 10 minutes and serve with extra salsa on the side.

Makes 4 servings

Per serving: 503 calories, 13 g fat, 25 mg cholesterol, 9 g fiber, 1,551 mg sodium

Barley-Corn Pilaf with Jack Cheese

You could also add ½ teaspoon of dried basil, dill, thyme, or other herb.

> 1   tablespoon butter or margarine
>
> 1   onion, finely chopped
>
> ½   cup finely chopped red bell pepper
>
> ¾   cup quick-cooking barley
>
> 1   can (14¾ ounces) fat-free, reduced-sodium chicken broth
>
> 1   can (11 ounces) corn kernels, drained
>
> ⅛   teaspoon freshly ground black pepper
>
> ½   cup shredded Monterey Jack cheese
>
> 1   tablespoon finely chopped parsley

1. Melt the butter or margarine in a medium saucepan over medium heat. Add the onion and cook for 3 minutes. Add the pepper. Cook for 3 minutes.

2. Stir in the barley, broth, corn, and black pepper. Bring to a boil. Reduce the heat to low, cover, and simmer for 15 to 18 minutes, or until the liquid is absorbed and the barley is tender.

3. Remove from the heat. Stir in the cheese and parsley. Cover and let stand for 5 minutes before serving.

Makes 6 servings

Per serving: 169 calories, 6 g fat, 14 mg cholesterol, 3 g fiber, 343 mg sodium

Pasta Shells in Broth with Tuna, White Beans, and Spinach

Substitute kale or collard greens for the spinach, if you like.

8	ounces small pasta shells
1	tablespoon olive oil
1	onion, finely chopped
4	cloves garlic, finely chopped
2	cans (14¾ ounces each) fat-free, reduced-sodium chicken broth
1	box (10 ounces) frozen chopped spinach, thawed and drained
½	teaspoon fennel seeds, crushed
¼	teaspoon salt (optional)
⅛	teaspoon freshly ground black pepper
1	can (15 ounces) navy or cannellini beans, rinsed and drained
1	can (6 ounces) water-packed tuna, drained and flaked
2	tablespoons lemon juice
½	cup grated Parmesan cheese (optional)

1. Cook the pasta according to package directions. Drain and return to the pot.

2. Warm the oil in a large saucepan over medium heat. Add the onion and cook for 3 minutes. Add the garlic and cook for 1 minute. Stir in the broth, spinach, fennel seeds, salt (if using), and pepper. Cook for 5 minutes. Stir in the beans, tuna, and lemon juice. Simmer for 2 minutes.

3. Add the pasta and stir to mix. Serve sprinkled with the cheese (if using).

Makes 4 servings

Per serving: 428 calories, 6 g fat, 13 mg cholesterol, 7 g fiber, 965 mg sodium

Potatoes Stuffed with Turkey Ham

This entrée is cooked in the microwave, so you can whip it up in no time flat.
For variety, use smoked turkey breast.

2	large baking potatoes
½	cup fat-free plain yogurt
1	cup chopped cooked turkey ham
½	cup finely chopped onion
½	cup finely chopped green pepper
¼	teaspoon freshly ground black pepper

1. Scrub the potatoes with cold water, then pat dry. Use a fork to prick the potatoes in several places. Place on a microwaveable plate and cover with plastic wrap. Vent the wrap by pulling back a small corner. Microwave on high power for 5 minutes. Rotate the plate a half-turn, then microwave on high power for 5 to 7 minutes, or until the potatoes are tender. Let stand, covered, for 5 minutes.

2. Cut each potato in half lengthwise. Scoop out the pulp (leaving ¼"-thick shells) and place the pulp in a medium bowl. Mash well with a potato masher. Stir in the yogurt. Then stir in the turkey ham, onions, green peppers, and black pepper.

3. Spoon the mixture into the potato shells. Transfer the shells to the plate and cover with plastic wrap. Vent the wrap. Microwave on high power for 3 to 4 minutes, or until heated through.

Makes 4 servings

Per serving: 118 calories, 2 g fat, 16 mg cholesterol, 2 g fiber, 311 mg sodium

Note: If you can spare the time and prefer your potatoes cooked in a conventional oven, bake them at 400°F for 40 to 60 minutes, or until tender.

You're angry.

What you need: healthy snack food

If you like your snacks crispy and crunchy, whip up one of these delicious low-fat recipes for chips, nachos, and dips for raw veggies. You can crunch and munch without guilt. You'll even find healthy recipes for two all-time favorites: pizza and peanut butter sandwiches.

COMMONSENSE STRATEGY:
If you crave crispy, crunchy foods when you're angry, these recipes are for you. But while they can satisfy your urge to bite off someone's head, consider trying tool 108 in the Mood Tools chapter first. It may help quell your desire to "eat yourself up" with anger.

Potato Chips

It's easy to make your own healthy chips. For nice thin ones, use a manual slicing machine (inexpensive plastic ones are available at cooking stores). For a gourmet touch, try blue or purple potatoes.

> 2 baking potatoes
> 2 sweet potatoes

1. Slice the potatoes as thinly as possible (about 20 slices per potato). Place 10 slices at a time on a microwaveable rack and microwave on high power for 4 minutes, or until golden and crispy.

2. Watch the first batch carefully. Microwaving time depends on the moisture content of the potatoes. If after 4 minutes the potatoes are not crisp, continue microwaving for 30 seconds at a time. Repeat to cook all the slices.

Makes 4 servings

Per serving: 66 calories, 0 g fat, 0 mg cholesterol, 2 g fiber, 5 mg sodium

Note: If you don't have a microwave, place a rack on a baking sheet. Arrange the potato slices on the rack. Bake at 450°F for 15 to 20 minutes, or until crisp.

Herbed Yogurt Cheese Dip

Serve the dip with raw vegetables or pretzels or use it as a spread on low-fat crackers.

2	cups fat-free plain yogurt (see note)
2	ounces reduced-fat cream cheese
1½	tablespoons finely chopped fresh chives
1	tablespoon finely chopped fresh basil
¼	teaspoon coarsely ground black pepper

1. Line a sieve with 2 layers of cheesecloth and set over a large bowl. Spoon the yogurt into the sieve. Cover and refrigerate for at least 12 hours, or until the yogurt is the consistency of cream cheese. You should have about 1 cup of yogurt cheese. Discard the liquid.

2. Place the yogurt cheese, cream cheese, chives, basil, and pepper in a food processor. Process until smooth. Spoon into a small bowl. Cover and refrigerate for at least 1 hour to allow the flavors to blend.

Makes 1 cup

Per 2 tablespoons: 42 calories, 2 g fat, 6 mg cholesterol, 0 g fiber, 54 mg sodium

Note: Use yogurt that does not contain gums as thickeners; they will prevent it from draining.

Light 'n' Lean Nachos

In this healthier version of this high-fat favorite, potatoes replace the traditional deep-fried tortilla chips. But eat your one portion—unless you're making them for company.

1½	pounds large potatoes, scrubbed and sliced crosswise ⅜" thick
½	cup fat-free, reduced-sodium chicken broth
1⅓	cups salsa
1	cup rinsed and drained canned pinto or white beans
½	teaspoon hot-pepper sauce
⅔	cup shredded reduced-fat Monterey Jack cheese

1. In a 4-cup glass measuring cup, combine half of the potatoes and ¼ cup of the broth. Cover with vented plastic wrap and microwave on high power for 5 to 7 minutes, or until the potatoes are just tender.

2. Let stand until cool enough to handle. Drain the potatoes and pat dry with paper towels. Spread on a large microwaveable serving plate.

3. In a small bowl, mix the salsa, beans, and hot-pepper sauce. Spoon half of the mixture over the potatoes. Sprinkle with ⅓ cup of the cheese. Loosely cover with waxed paper.

4. Microwave on medium power for 2 minutes, or until the cheese has melted. Serve immediately.

5. Repeat with the remaining potatoes, broth, salsa mixture, and cheese.

Makes 8 servings

Per serving: 146 calories, 3 g fat, 7 mg cholesterol, 2 g fiber, 215 mg sodium

Note: If you don't have a microwave, steam the potato slices until tender, about 10 minutes. Then spread them on ovenproof platters and top with the salsa mixture and cheese. Bake at 350°F for 15 minutes.

Fresh Tomato Salsa with Homemade Tortilla Chips

Goat cheese gives this traditional salsa an unexpected flavor twist. Enjoy it with these easy-to-make tortilla chips.

 1 **cup chopped plum tomatoes**
 ½ **cup chopped scallions**
 ½ **cup chopped fresh coriander**
 1 **tablespoon grated lime peel**
 1 **tablespoon lime juice**
 1 **teaspoon olive oil**
 ½ **jalapeño pepper, seeded and finely chopped (wear plastic gloves when handling)**
 1 **tablespoon crumbled goat cheese**
 4 **flour tortillas (12" diameter)**

1. Preheat the oven to 350°F. Coat a large baking sheet with cooking spray.

2. In a medium bowl, mix the tomatoes, scallions, coriander, lime peel, lime juice, oil, and peppers. Sprinkle with the cheese.

3. Cut each tortilla into 8 wedges. Place on the prepared baking sheet. Bake for 10 minutes, or until golden and crispy. Serve with the salsa.

Makes 8 servings

Per serving: 16 calories, 0.5 g fat, 0 mg cholesterol, 0 g fiber, 4 mg sodium

Grilled Peanut Butter and Banana Sandwich

This PB&B can be prepared just like a grilled cheese sandwich, although we've substituted light cooking spray for the pool of butter.

   6   tablespoons smooth or crunchy peanut butter
   8   slices whole grain bread
   2   large ripe bananas, sliced lengthwise into a total of 16 pieces
   2   tablespoons honey
       Butter-flavored cooking spray

1. Spread the peanut butter on the bread. Place the banana pieces on 4 of the slices and drizzle with the honey. Top with the remaining bread to make 4 sandwiches.

2. Place a large nonstick skillet over medium-high heat until hot. Coat the bread with cooking spray just before browning each side. Cook the sandwiches in batches for about 2 minutes per side, or until golden brown.

Makes 4 servings

Per serving: 357 calories, 14 g fat, 0 mg cholesterol, 6 g fiber, 322 mg sodium

---

HEALTHY PEANUT BUTTER SNACKS

Take a break from the old peanut butter and jelly routine. Instead, savor the flavors of these creative and oddly delicious fillings in peanut butter sandwiches. Start with creamy or chunky peanut butter and add:

Apple	Sliced fresh pears
Banana, dates, and honey	Raisins
Banana, lettuce, and ham	Raisins and carrots
Celery	Raisins and celery
Kiwifruit	Raisins and sunflower seeds

Vegetable Pizza with Goat Cheese

Here's a homemade pie that's in the oven in 10 minutes. The secret is precut vegetables, prepared pizza dough, and storebought pesto.

1	teaspoon cornmeal
1	package refrigerated pizza dough (1 pound)
2	tablespoons pesto
1	red onion, thinly sliced
1	large tomato, sliced
1	jar (7 ounces) roasted red bell peppers, drained
1	cup chopped broccoli florets
⅓	cup crumbled goat cheese
2	tablespoons grated Parmesan cheese

1. Preheat the oven to 500°F. Sprinkle the cornmeal on a large baking sheet.

2. Roll out the dough and place it on the sheet, pressing to fit. Spread with the pesto. Top with the onion and tomato. Sprinkle with the peppers, broccoli, goat cheese, and Parmesan cheese.

3. Bake for 10 to 15 minutes, or until the crust is browned and the cheese has melted.

Makes 4 servings

Per serving: 375 calories, 10 g fat, 11 mg cholesterol, 3 g fiber, 668 mg sodium

Chickpea Crunchies

These savory little nibbles are high in fiber, so they'll boost your intake at the same time that they satisfy your between-meal munchies.

1	cup canned chickpeas, rinsed and drained
1	tablespoon grated Parmesan cheese
1	teaspoon sour-cream-flavored granules
½	teaspoon curry powder
	Pinch of ground red pepper

1. Preheat the oven to 350°F. Coat an 8" round baking pan with cooking spray.
2. Pat the chickpeas dry with paper towels. In a medium bowl, stir together the cheese, granules, curry powder, and pepper. Add the chickpeas and toss to coat well.
3. Transfer to the prepared pan. Bake, stirring every 5 minutes, for 30 minutes, or until dry and golden. Cool completely and store in an airtight container.

Makes 1 cup

Per ¼ cup: 55 calories, 1.5 g fat, 1 mg cholesterol, 2 g fiber, 232 mg sodium

Crispy Wonton Chips

These chips are so low in fat and calories that you can munch on them without feeling guilty. The wonton wrappers store well in the refrigerator or freezer. For variety, sprinkle the wrappers with ground red pepper or chili powder before baking.

30	wonton wrappers (3" square)

1. Preheat the oven to 350°F. Coat 2 large baking sheets with cooking spray. Arrange the wonton wrappers in a single layer on the sheets.
2. Coat the wonton wrappers with cooking spray. Using a pizza cutter or sharp knife, cut each diagonally in half. Bake for 5 minutes, or until lightly brown and crisp.

Makes 60

Per 6 chips: 42 calories, 0.5 g fat, 0 mg cholesterol, 0 g fiber, 0 mg sodium

Chili-Cheese Popcorn

Add the Parmesan seasoning mixture while the popcorn is still hot so the cheese melts slightly and sticks to the popcorn. Use homemade air-popped corn because it has no added fat.

1½–2 tablespoons grated Parmesan cheese
½–1 teaspoon chili powder
¼ teaspoon dried oregano or marjoram
14 cups hot air-popped popcorn

1. In a custard cup, mix the cheese, chili powder, and oregano or marjoram.
2. Place the hot popcorn in a large bowl and quickly toss it with the cheese mixture.

Makes 14 cups

Per 1 cup: 29 calories, 0.5 g fat, 0 mg cholesterol, 1 g fiber, 13 mg sodium

Barbecued Popcorn

When chips seem to be calling your name, whip up a batch of this savory popcorn that's way lower in fat but still crunchy and slightly salty.

2 tablespoons molasses
2 tablespoons reduced-sodium barbecue sauce
1 tablespoon reduced-sodium ketchup
½ teaspoon paprika
½ teaspoon garlic powder
8 cups air-popped popcorn

1. Preheat the oven to 200°F. Line a large baking sheet with foil and coat with cooking spray.
2. In a small bowl, mix the molasses, barbecue sauce, ketchup, paprika, and garlic powder. Place the popcorn in a large bowl. Drizzle with the molasses mixture. Toss well to coat.
3. Spread the popcorn mixture on the prepared baking sheet. Bake for 20 minutes. Turn off the oven and let the popcorn cool in the oven for 30 minutes, or until crisp.

Makes 8 cups

Per 1 cup: 50 calories, 0 g fat, 0 mg cholesterol, 1 g fiber, 35 mg sodium

You're stressed.

What you need: comfort food

Even when you're under stress, you still need to eat. But don't turn to takeout for comfort. These savory but slimmed-down dishes—meat loaf, mashed potatoes, hot-fudge sundaes—will remind you of the meals Mom used to make. And that can make anyone feel better.

COMMONSENSE STRATEGY: Go ahead . . . splurge on these comfort foods. But before you've enjoyed your one serving, freeze the rest, give it away—or throw it out, if need be. Scarfing five or six servings instead of one will make you feel guilty and stress you out even more.

Mashed Potatoes

These mashed potatoes are as creamy as the ones Mom used to make. Low-fat milk and fat-free sour cream replace the traditional butter and whole milk.

1½	pounds potatoes, peeled and cubed
1½	teaspoons trans-free tub-style margarine
1½	teaspoons butter-flavored sprinkles
¼	cup fat-free sour cream
½–¾	cup 1% milk, warmed
½	teaspoon salt
¼	teaspoon freshly ground black pepper
¼	teaspoon paprika

1. Place the potatoes in a large saucepan and cover with cold water. Bring to a boil over medium-high heat. Boil for 15 minutes, or until the potatoes are tender when pierced with a fork. Drain well.

2. Return the potatoes to the pan. Add the margarine and butter-flavored sprinkles. Using a potato masher or hand-held electric mixer, mash the potatoes thoroughly. Beat in the sour cream and enough of the milk to achieve a creamy consistency. Beat in the salt, pepper, and paprika.

Makes 4 servings

Per serving: 169 calories, 2 g fat, 1 mg cholesterol, 0 g fiber, 341 mg sodium

Turkey Pot Pie with Buttermilk Biscuit Crust

Cooked turkey and frozen mixed vegetables streamline this family favorite.

1	cup all-purpose flour
1	teaspoon baking powder
¼	teaspoon baking soda
	Pinch of salt
1	tablespoon + 2 teaspoons chilled butter, cut into small pieces
¼	cup low-fat buttermilk
3	tablespoons reduced-fat sour cream
1¾	cups fat-free, reduced-sodium chicken broth
⅓	cup chopped onion
2	teaspoons finely chopped garlic
2½	tablespoons cornstarch
¼	teaspoon poultry seasoning
½	teaspoon dried thyme
¼	teaspoon dried sage
2	cups frozen mixed peas, carrots, and cauliflower, thawed
2	cups diced cooked turkey breast

1. Preheat the oven to 425°F.

2. In a medium bowl, mix the flour, baking powder, baking soda, and salt. Cut in the butter with 2 knives until the mixture resembles fine crumbs. Stir in the buttermilk and sour cream to form a dough. Turn the dough onto a sheet of plastic wrap and flatten it into a large disk. Wrap tightly. Refrigerate while you make the filling.

3. Bring ¼ cup of the broth to a boil in a large skillet. Add the onion and garlic. Cook for 2 minutes.

4. In a small bowl, mix the cornstarch, poultry seasoning, thyme, and sage. Stir in the remaining 1½ cups broth until smooth. Add to the pan. Cook until the mixture comes to a boil and thickens. Remove from the heat and add the vegetables and turkey. Pour into an 8" × 8" baking dish.

5. Cut the biscuit dough into four sections. Arrange on top of the filling. Bake for 30 minutes, or until the biscuits are golden brown and the filling is bubbling.

Makes 4 servings

Per serving: 331 calories, 7 g fat, 64 mg cholesterol, 3 g fiber, 536 mg sodium

Spicy Chicken Noodle Soup

Food doesn't get any more comforting than this—whether you're tired, chilled, or coming down with a cold.

1   **package (9 ounces) fresh angel hair pasta**

6   **cups fat-free, reduced-sodium chicken broth**

3   **cups water**

6   **cloves garlic, coarsely chopped**

1   **piece fresh ginger (1½" long), unpeeled and cut into 3 pieces**

3   **dried small hot red peppers**

½   **pound skinless, boneless chicken breast, cut into bite-size pieces**

4   **scallions, finely chopped**

1. Place the pasta in a large heatproof bowl. Pour enough boiling water over the pasta to cover it. Stir gently with a fork to break up the noodles. Set aside.

2. In a large saucepan, combine the broth, water, garlic, ginger, and peppers. Bring to a boil over high heat. Reduce the heat to low and simmer for 10 minutes. Add the chicken and cook for 5 minutes, or until the chicken is no longer pink in the center when cut in half.

3. Drain the noodles and add to the saucepan. Cook, stirring with a fork, for 1 to 2 minutes. Stir in the scallions. Remove and discard the ginger and peppers.

Makes 6 servings

Per serving: 198 calories, 4 g fat, 28 mg cholesterol, 2 g fiber, 274 mg sodium

All-American Meat Loaf

Here's a moist meat loaf that boasts great flavor and is good for you, too.

2 cups shredded cabbage

1 cup chopped onion

1 cup shredded carrot

½ cup chopped green pepper

2 cloves garlic, finely chopped

1 cup cooked brown rice or barley

1 teaspoon dried basil

½ teaspoon dried savory

¼ teaspoon dried thyme

1 pound extra-lean ground beef

3 egg whites, lightly beaten

¾ teaspoon salt

¼ teaspoon freshly ground black pepper

Horseradish mustard

1. Preheat the oven to 350°F. Coat a 9" × 5" loaf pan with cooking spray.

2. Coat a large skillet with cooking spray and warm over medium heat. Add the cabbage, onion, carrot, green pepper, and garlic. Cover and cook, stirring occasionally, for 8 to 10 minutes, or until the carrot is tender. Stir in the rice or barley, basil, savory, and thyme. Let cool for 5 to 10 minutes.

3. Add the beef, egg whites, salt, and black pepper. Mix with your hands to combine. Pack the mixture into the prepared loaf pan.

4. Bake for 1 hour. Let cool for 5 minutes. Turn onto a platter and slice. Serve with the horseradish mustard.

Makes 6 servings

Per serving: 165 calories, 7 g fat, 35 mg cholesterol, 2 g fiber, 261 mg sodium

Guilt-Free Macaroni and Cheese

To cut fat (more than 50 percent!) without losing flavor, start with flavorful ingredients. We used extra-sharp Cheddar cheese and Dijon mustard for maximum flavor and pureed cottage cheese for extra creaminess.

6	ounces elbow macaroni
1½	teaspoons butter or trans-free margarine
1	small onion, finely chopped
1	tablespoon all-purpose flour
1	cup 1% milk
¼	teaspoon salt
⅛	teaspoon pepper
3	ounces grated extra-sharp Cheddar cheese
8	ounces 1% cottage cheese
1	teaspoon Dijon mustard
2	tablespoons grated Parmesan cheese
2	tablespoons dried bread crumbs

1. Preheat the oven to 375°F. Coat an 8" × 8" baking dish with cooking spray.

2. Cook the macaroni according to package directions. Drain and rinse with cool water, then drain again.

3. Melt the butter or margarine in a medium saucepan. Add the onion and cook for 5 minutes or until soft. Sprinkle with the flour and stir well. Gradually stir in the milk, salt, and pepper. Cook over medium heat, stirring often, for 10 minutes, or until slightly thickened. Remove from the heat and stir in the Cheddar cheese.

4. Process the cottage cheese and mustard in a blender until smooth. Gradually stir into the cheese sauce. Add the macaroni and spoon into the prepared baking dish. Combine the Parmesan cheese and bread crumbs. Sprinkle evenly over the macaroni mixture.

5. Bake for 35 minutes or until bubbly.

Makes 4 servings

Per serving: 170 calories, 5.5 g fat, 17 mg cholesterol, 0 g fiber, 311 mg sodium

Quiche Florentine

We've reduced the fat of traditional quiche by replacing the pastry crust with bread crumbs and using reduced-fat cheeses and fat-free evaporated milk.

3 tablespoons unseasoned dry bread crumbs

1 tablespoon finely chopped parsley

1 cup sliced mushrooms

2 tablespoons chopped onion

¼ teaspoon dried thyme

5 ounces frozen spinach, thawed and squeezed dry

1 tablespoon all-purpose flour

⅓ cup reduced-fat cottage cheese

¼ cup shredded reduced-fat Swiss cheese

1 can (12 ounces) fat-free evaporated milk

3 eggs

⅛ teaspoon ground nutmeg

¼ teaspoon salt

¼ teaspoon freshly ground black pepper

1. Preheat the oven to 350°F. Coat a 9" pie plate with cooking spray. In a small bowl, mix together the bread crumbs and parsley. Sprinkle evenly over the bottom and sides of the pie plate.

2. Coat a large skillet with cooking spray and warm over medium heat. Add the mushrooms, onion, and thyme. Cover and cook for 3 minutes, or until the mushrooms are soft.

3. Add the spinach to the skillet and cook, uncovered, for 3 to 4 minutes, or until the mixture is quite dry. Stir in the flour and cook for 1 minute. Remove from the heat and stir in the cottage cheese and Swiss cheese.

4. In a medium bowl, beat together the milk, eggs, nutmeg, salt, and pepper. Stir in the spinach mixture. Pour into the prepared pie plate.

5. Bake for 35 minutes, or until the quiche is lightly browned and a knife inserted in the center comes out clean. Cool on a rack for 5 minutes.

Makes 4 servings

Per serving: 216 calories, 6 g fat, 168 mg cholesterol, 1 g fiber, 440 mg sodium

Hot-Fudge Sundaes

A dieter's dream come true—the guilt-free sundae!

- 1 tablespoon unsweetened cocoa powder
- 1 tablespoon reduced-calorie maple-flavored syrup
- 2 teaspoons cornstarch
- ⅓ cup water
- ½ teaspoon vanilla extract
- 1 cup frozen low-fat vanilla yogurt

1. In a small saucepan, stir together the cocoa powder, maple syrup, and cornstarch until smooth. Stir in the water.

2. Bring the mixture to a boil over medium-high heat, stirring constantly. Reduce the heat to medium. Stir for 1 minute, or until the mixture slightly thickens. Remove from the heat and stir in the vanilla. Serve hot over the frozen yogurt.

Makes 2 servings

Per serving: 112 calories, 0.5 g fat, 0 mg cholesterol, 0 g fiber, 31 mg sodium

Strawberries with Creamy Banana Sauce

Pureed bananas make a wonderfully rich, creamy sauce that you can serve over other fruit (or even over angel food cake). Just be sure to serve the sauce soon after it's made, otherwise the bananas will turn brown.

- ½ cup fat-free plain yogurt
- ⅓ banana, thickly sliced
- ½ teaspoon honey
- ¼ teaspoon vanilla extract
- 2 cups halved strawberries

1. Place the yogurt, banana, honey, and vanilla in a blender. Process until smooth. Spoon over the strawberries.

Makes 4 servings

Per serving: 51 calories, 0.5 g fat, 1 mg cholesterol, 2 g fiber, 23 mg sodium

New-Wave Streusel Apples

When you need a fast dessert to satisfy a sweet craving,
try this sweet but healthy treat.

¼ **cup fat-free plain yogurt**

1 **tablespoon honey**

2 **medium cooking apples (see note)**

2 **tablespoons quick-cooking oats**

1 **tablespoon brown sugar**

1 **tablespoon reduced-calorie trans-free margarine, softened**

½ **teaspoon ground cinnamon**

1. In a small bowl, mix the yogurt and honey.

2. Core the apples to within ½" of the bottom. Peel the top third of each apple.

3. In a small bowl, mix the oats, brown sugar, margarine, and cinnamon. Spoon into the centers of the apples.

4. Place the apples in a small microwaveable dish. Microwave on high power for 6 minutes, or until the apples are nearly tender. Rotate the dish a half-turn after 3 minutes. Cover with plastic wrap and let stand for 3 minutes to finish cooking.

5. To serve, cut each apple lengthwise in half. Top with the yogurt mixture.

Makes 4 servings

Per serving: 110 calories, 2 g fat, 0 mg cholesterol, 2 g fiber, 45 mg sodium

Note: Cooking apples—like Cortland, Granny Smith, Rome Beauty, Winesap, and York—hold their shape well when baked and are a better choice than McIntosh, Empire, and other varieties that turn soft and mushy quickly.

Cranberry-Peach Compote

We reduced calories in this compote by cooking the fruit in juice rather than the conventional sugar syrup. If you like, top each serving with a spoonful of fat-free vanilla yogurt or a scoop of fat-free frozen yogurt.

- 1 cup orange juice
- ½ cup pineapple juice
- 2 tablespoons honey
- 1 tablespoon grated orange peel
- 1 tablespoon grated fresh ginger
- ½ teaspoon ground cinnamon
- ¼ teaspoon ground nutmeg
- 2 cups cranberries
- ½ cup golden raisins
- 8 dried apricot halves
- 1 can (16 ounces) sliced peaches (packed in juice)

1. In a medium saucepan, combine the orange juice, pineapple juice, honey, orange peel, ginger, cinnamon, and nutmeg. Bring to a boil over high heat. Stir in the cranberries, raisins, and apricots. Reduce the heat to medium-low and simmer for 10 to 12 minutes, or until the cranberries begin to pop.

2. Place the peaches in a medium bowl. Pour the hot cranberry mixture over the peaches and gently stir just until combined. Cover and refrigerate for at least 4 hours.

Makes 8 servings

Per serving: 119 calories, 0.5 g fat, 0 mg cholesterol, 1 g fiber, 5 mg sodium

You work at home . . . and the refrigerator beckons.

What you need: healthy sandwiches and nukeable, make-ahead meals

When your work is at home, the kitchen is always open. The key: Fill your fridge with washed, cut-up veggies and fruit. Don't eat at your desk. Eat at the dining-room table. (The only paper you see should be a napkin.) And finally, enjoy these healthy, simple sandwiches, salads, and veggie-based dishes.

COMMONSENSE STRATEGY: Most of these recipes yield 4 to 6 servings. When you prepare them, immediately divide into single-serving portions and freeze.

Store prepared salads and veggies in plastic containers clearly labeled "lunch."

Rosemary Roasted Vegetables

They're an outstanding accompaniment to chicken breasts, fish fillets, and turkey burgers.

2   red bell peppers, quartered

2   medium onions, quartered

2   zucchini, cut into 2" pieces

1   tablespoon olive oil

1   teaspoon chopped fresh rosemary

1   teaspoon finely chopped garlic

1   teaspoon balsamic vinegar

    Salt

    Freshly ground black pepper

1. Preheat the oven to 400°F.

2. Place the red peppers, onion, and zucchini on a broiler pan. Drizzle with the oil and toss lightly to coat. Spread in an even layer. Roast for 30 minutes.

3. Sprinkle with the rosemary, garlic, and vinegar. Toss lightly.

Makes 4 servings

Per serving: 85 calories, 4 g fat, 0 mg cholesterol, 4 g fiber, 0 mg sodium

Ricotta, Feta, and Spinach Pie

This creamy cheese-and-spinach pie tastes decadent but isn't.
So go on—indulge!

1	tablespoon dried bread crumbs
1	bag (10 ounces) fresh spinach
1	cup reduced-fat ricotta cheese
3	large eggs
½	cup fat-free half-and-half
⅓	cup crumbled feta cheese
¾	teaspoon finely chopped garlic
½	teaspoon salt
¼	teaspoon freshly ground black pepper
	Pinch of grated nutmeg

1. Preheat the oven to 350°F. Coat a 9" pie plate with nonstick spray. Sprinkle with the bread crumbs to coat.

2. Cook the spinach according to package directions. Cool, then squeeze out the excess liquid. Coarsely chop.

3. In a large bowl, mix the ricotta cheese, eggs, half-and-half, feta cheese, garlic, salt, pepper, and nutmeg. Stir in the spinach. Pour into the prepared pie plate, smooth the top, and bake for 35 minutes, or until the top is lightly puffed and rounded. Let stand for 5 minutes before cutting.

Makes 4 servings

Per serving: 148 calories, 8 g fat, 176 mg cholesterol, 2 g fiber, 608 mg sodium

Spicy Beans and Greens

Ladle this main dish into a bowl and enjoy with crusty whole wheat Italian
bread. Greens never tasted this hearty.

1	tablespoon olive oil
2	large onions, chopped
2	tablespoons finely chopped garlic
3	cups canned cannellini or white beans, rinsed and drained
1¼	cups fat-free, reduced-sodium chicken broth

¼ teaspoon salt

1 pound Swiss chard, washed and trimmed

½ teaspoon red-pepper flakes

1. Warm the oil in a large skillet over medium heat. Add the onion and garlic and cook, stirring occasionally, for 5 minutes, or until the onion is soft.

2. Add the beans, broth, and salt. Bring to a boil. Reduce the heat and simmer for 5 minutes.

3. Stir in the Swiss chard and red-pepper flakes. Simmer for 1 minute.

Makes 4 servings

Per serving: 314 calories, 4 g fat, 0 mg cholesterol, 3 g fiber, 911 mg sodium

Pear and Smoked Turkey Salad

It's amazing how well smoked turkey complements fresh pears. Serve this salad as lunch or an appetizer at dinner.

4 Anjou or Bartlett pears

2 ounces thinly sliced smoked turkey breast

2 tablespoons rice vinegar or white-wine vinegar

4 teaspoons olive oil

1 tablespoon honey

2 tablespoons finely chopped fresh basil

Freshly ground black pepper

1. Quarter the pears lengthwise and remove the cores. Cut each quarter in half lengthwise. Arrange the pears decoratively on a platter, alternating occasionally with strips of smoked turkey.

2. In a small bowl, whisk the vinegar, oil, and honey until smooth. Stir in the basil. Spoon over the pears and turkey. Season lightly with the pepper.

Makes 4 servings

Per serving: 190 calories, 5.5 g fat, 4 mg cholesterol, 5 g fiber, 151 mg sodium

Mexican Tuna Cobb Salad

Accompany the salad with low-fat oven-baked tortilla chips or warm corn tortillas—and be sure everyone gets a good look at this impressive salad before you dish it out.

Dressing

¼ cup chopped fresh cilantro
¼ cup fat-free mayonnaise
¼ cup fat-free plain yogurt
3 tablespoons drained canned chopped green chile peppers
2 tablespoons finely chopped red onion
2 tablespoons lime juice
1 teaspoon grated lime peel
¼ teaspoon salt
⅛ teaspoon freshly ground black pepper

Salad

8 cups Romaine lettuce, thinly sliced
1 can (19 ounces) pinto or red kidney beans, rinsed and drained
1 can (6 ounces) water-packed tuna, drained and flaked
4 plum tomatoes, diced
1 small cucumber, peeled, seeded, and diced
1 medium yellow or red bell pepper, diced
½ medium avocado, peeled and diced
½ cup diced radishes

1. *To make the dressing:* In a small bowl, mix the cilantro, mayonnaise, yogurt, chile peppers, onion, lime juice, lime peel, salt, and pepper.

2. *To make the salad:* Place the lettuce in a large bowl. Add ¼ cup of the dressing and toss well. Arrange the lettuce on a platter.

3. Spoon the beans, tuna, tomatoes, cucumber, pepper, avocado, radishes, and some of the dressing in parallel rows on top of the lettuce. Place the remaining dressing in a small bowl to serve on the side.

Makes 4 servings

Per serving: 231 calories, 5.5 g fat, 17 mg cholesterol, 8 g fiber, 668 mg sodium

Vegetables on the Grill

Grilling is such a simple way to prepare vegetables and brings out their best flavors. You can also prepare these vegetables under the broiler. Cook them 4" to 6" from the heat for 5 to 8 minutes.

2	small zucchini, sliced diagonally ¼" thick
2	small yellow summer squash, sliced diagonally ¼" thick
2	small eggplant, sliced diagonally ¼" thick
1	red bell pepper, halved lengthwise and seeded
2	red onions, sliced crosswise ⅜" thick
¼	teaspoon freshly ground black pepper
	Pinch of salt

1. Preheat the grill.

2. Coat an unheated grill rack with olive oil cooking spray. Arrange the zucchini, yellow squash, eggplant, red peppers, and onions on the rack and coat lightly with the spray.

3. Place the rack over medium-hot coals, arranging it so the vegetables are 6" from the coals. Grill for 4 to 6 minutes on each side, or until the vegetables turn golden brown. Sprinkle with the black pepper and salt.

Makes 6 servings

Per serving: 49 calories, 0.5 g fat, 0 mg cholesterol, 8 g fiber, 5 mg sodium

Grilled Vegetable Sandwich

This fast focaccia sandwich is perfect for a summer lunch with a side salad and a fruit dessert. You can also cook the vegetables under the broiler.

1	large red bell pepper, quartered lengthwise and seeded
½	tablespoon olive oil
½	onion, thinly sliced
½	cup sliced mushrooms
1	large clove garlic, finely chopped
⅛	teaspoon fennel seeds
	Salt (optional)
	Freshly ground black pepper
1	square (4") thick focaccia bread

1. Preheat the grill.

2. Lightly coat the red pepper with cooking spray and grill, turning frequently, for 5 to 6 minutes, or until lightly browned. Cool slightly and cut into strips.

3. Coat a large skillet with cooking spray and warm over medium heat. Add the oil, onion, mushrooms, garlic, and fennel seeds. Cook for 10 minutes, or until the vegetables soften and turn golden.

4. Add the pepper slices. Cook for 2 to 3 minutes, or until heated through. Season with the salt (if using) and black pepper.

5. Split the focaccia bread horizontally and fill with the vegetable mixture.

Makes 1 serving

Per serving: 282 calories, 7 g fat, 0 mg cholesterol, 5 g fiber, 293 mg sodium

Savory Cheese Pockets

Here's a breakfast sandwich that can also double as a slimming brown-bag lunch entrée.

 1 **cup 1% cottage cheese**
 1 **tablespoon fat-free milk**
 ½ **cup shredded zucchini**
 ¼ **cup shredded reduced-fat Cheddar cheese**
 ½ **teaspoon dried dillweed**
 ¼ **teaspoon onion powder**
 2 **whole wheat pitas**

1. In a blender, process the cottage cheese and milk until smooth. Transfer to a small bowl. Stir in the zucchini, Cheddar cheese, dillweed, and onion powder.

2. Cut each pita crosswise in half to form 2 pockets. Fill each pocket with the cheese mixture.

Makes 4 servings

Per serving: 222 calories, 3.5 g fat, 13 mg cholesterol, 1 g fiber, 906 mg sodium

Note: You can make these sandwiches ahead and freeze for quick breakfasts or carry-along lunches. Individually wrap each sandwich in freezer wrap and freeze. Thaw overnight in the refrigerator or pack the frozen sandwich in a lunch bag (it will thaw by lunchtime).

Pitas Stuffed with Chicken-Apple Salad

The combination of chicken and fruit is particularly appealing. Serve these sandwiches for a light lunch in the middle of summer.

2	cups cubed cooked chicken breast
2	red apples, chopped
1	can (8 ounces) crushed pineapple (packed in juice), drained
½	cup chopped celery
⅓	cup low-fat lemon yogurt
¼	cup fat-free mayonnaise
¼	teaspoon celery seeds
4	whole wheat pitas
4	lettuce leaves

1. In a medium bowl, mix the chicken, apples, pineapple, and celery.

2. In a small bowl, mix the yogurt, mayonnaise, and celery seeds. Add to the chicken mixture and toss well.

3. Cut the top from each pita. Line each pita with a lettuce leaf and spoon in about 1 cup of the chicken mixture.

Makes 4 servings

Per serving: 346 calories, 6.5 g fat, 63 mg cholesterol, 3 g fiber, 493 mg sodium

Note: This sandwich filling is best served within 2 hours. If it stands longer, the acid in the pineapple will tend to soften the chicken.

Tuna and Zucchini Melts

Here's a lighter update of an old classic. The zucchini boosts the sandwich's fiber content and adds extra crunch to the filling.

- 1   can (9¼ ounces) water-packed tuna, drained and flaked
- ½   cup fat-free mayonnaise
- ¼   cup finely chopped celery
- ¼   cup shredded zucchini
- 2   scallions, thinly sliced
- 1   teaspoon mustard
- ¼   cup shredded reduced-fat Cheddar cheese
- 4   English muffins, split and toasted
- 8   tomato slices

1. Preheat the broiler.

2. In a medium bowl, mix the tuna, mayonnaise, celery, zucchini, scallions, and mustard. Stir in the cheese.

3. Spread about ¼ cup of the mixture on each English muffin half. Place the muffins on a baking sheet or broiler pan. Broil 3" to 4" from the heat for 4 minutes, or until the tuna mixture is heated through. Top each muffin with a tomato slice and broil for 1 to 2 minutes, or until the tomatoes are heated through.

Makes 4 servings

Per serving: 260 calories, 3.5 g fat, 26 mg cholesterol, 2 g fiber, 822 mg sodium

The holiday season has begun.

What you need: healthy holiday fare

What's Independence Day without burgers, Thanksgiving without candied sweet potatoes, Passover without charoset? No need to give them up. Here, you'll find lighter versions of traditional Easter, Thanksgiving, Passover, and Christmas dinners, as well as Fourth of July favorites. And that's something to celebrate.

COMMONSENSE STRATEGY: While these holiday recipes are wonderfully healthy, it can't hurt to take out some "leftovers life insurance." If you can't or don't want to freeze the leftovers, wrap them up and give them to your guests to take home.

Fourth of July

Come summer, picnics are the order of the day. And what fun is the Fourth of July celebration without burgers, corn, potato salad, and a selection of summer-fresh desserts? Don't let your diet go to the dogs during the dog days; just lighten it with dishes like these.

Zesty Cantaloupe Salad

The lime juice, pepper, and mint zest up this mellow-flavored fruit.

 1   medium cantaloupe
 1   small jalapeño pepper, seeded and finely minced (wear plastic gloves when handling)
 2   tablespoons fresh lime juice
 1   tablespoon minced fresh mint
 ⅛   teaspoon salt

1. Cut the cantaloupe in half. Scoop out and discard the seeds. Cut each half into 6 wedges. Peel and cut into ½-inch pieces. Place in a medium bowl.

2. Add the pepper, lime juice, mint, and salt. Stir to mix.

Makes 4 servings

Per serving: 56 calories, 0.4 g fat, 0 mg cholesterol, 1.4 g fiber, 83 mg sodium

Spinach Turkey Burgers with Corn Salsa

These tasty burgers have a fraction of the fat in regular ones but the same great flavor. Serve on whole grain rolls. The corn salsa has such a fresh flavor you won't even consider adding fatty extras to the burgers. When tomatoes and corn are out of season, use 1 can (14½ ounces) cut tomatoes and 1 can (11 ounces) corn kernels.

Burgers

1 pound ground turkey breast

1 package (10 ounces) frozen chopped spinach, thawed and well drained (see note)

1 medium onion, grated

½ cup instant oatmeal

1 egg white

½ teaspoon dried sage or oregano

½ teaspoon salt

Pinch of freshly ground black pepper

Salsa

2 cups chopped tomatoes

1½ cups cooked fresh corn kernels

1 scallion, finely chopped

1 tablespoon finely chopped cilantro

Salt

Freshly ground black pepper

1. *To make the burgers:* Preheat the grill or broiler.

2. In a medium bowl, mix the turkey, spinach, onion, oatmeal, egg white, sage or oregano, salt, and pepper. Shape into 4 patties. Cook for 6 to 8 minutes per side, or until browned and cooked through.

3. *To make the salsa:* In a medium bowl, mix the tomatoes, corn, scallion, and cilantro. Add salt and pepper to taste. Serve with the burgers.

Makes 4 servings

Per serving: 275 calories, 3.5 g fat, 66 mg cholesterol, 8 g fiber, 513 mg sodium

Note: Thaw the spinach in the microwave oven according to package directions. Cool slightly, then squeeze out excess liquid with your hands.

Creamy Potato Salad

Green beans and olives give this picnic favorite an intriguing new character.

2½ pounds small red-skinned potatoes
1¾ teaspoons salt
¾ pound green beans, cut to 1" pieces
⅓ cup water
½ cup reduced-fat mayonnaise
½ cup fat-free sour cream
1 tablespoon Dijon mustard
1 tablespoon cider vinegar
½ teaspoon freshly ground black pepper
¼ cup chopped pitted Greek olives, such as kalamata
2 tablespoons diced celery
2 tablespoons finely chopped onion

1. Place the potatoes in a large saucepan. Add 1½ teaspoons of the salt and cold water to cover by 2". Bring to a boil. Simmer over medium heat for 10 to 15 minutes, or until the potatoes are fork-tender. Drain well. Let cool slightly, then peel and cut into ¾" cubes.

2. In a microwaveable bowl, combine the beans and water. Cover and microwave on high power for 5 to 6 minutes, or until crisp-tender. Drain.

3. In a large bowl, mix the mayonnaise, sour cream, mustard, vinegar, pepper, and the remaining ¼ teaspoon salt. Stir in the potatoes, beans, olives, celery, and onion. Cover and chill.

Makes about 8 cups

Per ½ cup: 95 calories, 2 g fat, 0 mg cholesterol, 2 g fiber, 198 mg sodium

Broiled Vegetable Kebabs

Here's a meatless kebab that'll fool even meat lovers. The soy sauce in the marinade gives the tofu cubes a light tan color similar to pork or veal.

12	ounces firm tofu, cut into 1" cubes
1	medium yellow summer squash, cut into 1" pieces
16	cherry tomatoes
16	radishes
1	green bell pepper, cut into 1" pieces
¾	cup pineapple juice
1	tablespoon lime juice
1	tablespoon reduced-sodium soy sauce
2	cloves garlic, crushed
¼	teaspoon ground allspice
	Pinch of ground red pepper
2	cups hot cooked brown rice

1. Coat a large skillet with cooking spray and warm over medium heat. Add the tofu and cook for 4 to 5 minutes, or until golden on all sides, stirring frequently. Transfer to a large bowl. Add the squash, tomatoes, radishes, and green pepper.

2. In a small bowl, mix the pineapple juice, lime juice, soy sauce, garlic, allspice, and red pepper. Pour over the tofu mixture and gently toss until coated. Marinate at room temperature for at least 15 minutes to blend the flavors.

3. Preheat the broiler. Coat the rack of a broiling pan with cooking spray.

4. Drain the tofu mixture, reserving the marinade. Alternately thread the tofu and vegetables onto 8 skewers. Place the kebabs on the rack and brush with the reserved marinade. Broil 3" to 4" from the heat for 8 to 10 minutes, or until the vegetables are tender, brushing with any of the remaining marinade and turning frequently. Serve over the rice.

Makes 4 servings

Per serving: 293 calories, 9 g fat, 0 mg cholesterol, 5 g fiber, 179 mg sodium

Note: To keep tofu sweet and fresh, store it in the refrigerator immersed in water. Change the water every other day. The tofu will last up to 2 weeks.

Cherry-Peach Crisp

What better use for the season's tree-ripe peaches and cherries!

4	cups sliced peaches (see note)
2	cups pitted dark sweet cherries (see note)
½	cup + 2 tablespoons sugar
4	tablespoons flour
½	teaspoon ground ginger
¼	teaspoon ground nutmeg
⅛	teaspoon salt
1¾	cups low-fat granola
3	tablespoons butter or trans-free margarine, melted

1. Preheat the oven to 375°F. Coat a shallow 1½-quart baking dish with cooking spray.

2. In a medium bowl, mix the peaches, cherries, ½ cup sugar, 3 tablespoons flour, ginger, ⅛ teaspoon nutmeg, and salt. Pour into the baking dish.

3. In a medium bowl, mix the granola, butter or margarine, remaining 2 tablespoons sugar, remaining 1 tablespoon flour, and remaining ⅛ teaspoon nutmeg. Sprinkle over the peach mixture.

4. Bake for 35 to 40 minutes, or until the filling is bubbling and the top is browned. (If the top browns too quickly, cover loosely with foil and continue baking.) Serve warm or at room temperature.

Makes 8 servings

Per serving: 249 calories, 6 g fat, 12 mg cholesterol, 3 g fiber, 104 mg sodium

Note: Out of season, use 1 bag (20 ounces) frozen peach slices and 1 bag (12 ounces) frozen pitted dark sweet cherries. Thaw the fruit before using and toss with 1 tablespoon cornstarch.

Coconut Fool

A fool is a great old-fashioned dessert.

½   cup sweetened shredded coconut

2   pints strawberries, quartered

2   bananas, sliced

2   teaspoons grated orange peel

¾   cup fat-free whipped topping

¾   cup reduced-fat sour cream

1   tablespoon brown sugar

1. Preheat the oven to 350°F. Spread the coconut in a thin layer on a baking sheet. Bake, stirring occasionally, for 10 minutes, or until lightly browned. Let cool about 5 minutes.

2. In a large bowl, mix the strawberries and bananas. Fold in the orange peel, whipped topping, sour cream, brown sugar, and 6 tablespoons of the coconut. Divide among 4 serving bowls. Sprinkle with the remaining 2 tablespoons coconut.

Makes 4 servings

Per serving: 237 calories, 8 g fat, 0 mg cholesterol, 5 g fiber, 43 mg sodium

Fresh Fruit Tart with Olive Oil Crust

Substituting oil for butter in the crust reduces the saturated fat without sacrificing flavor.

1½   cups all-purpose flour

1   tablespoon + ½ cup sugar

½   teaspoon + ⅛ teaspoon salt

5   tablespoons light (or regular) olive oil

½   teaspoon white vinegar

2   tablespoons water

1½   cups 1% milk

1   egg

¼   cup cornstarch

½   cup fat-free half-and-half

1   teaspoon vanilla extract

4   small apricots, pitted and sliced into thin wedges

2   kiwifruit, peeled and sliced into thin half-rounds

½   cup fresh raspberries

1. Preheat the oven to 400°F. Coat a 10½" tart pan with cooking spray.

2. In a medium bowl, mix the flour, 1 tablespoon sugar, and ½ teaspoon salt. Stir in the oil and vinegar with a fork until well combined. Add the water, stirring until the dough holds together.

3. Shape the dough into a disk and roll between 2 sheets of plastic wrap into a 12½" circle. Freeze on a baking sheet for 15 minutes. Remove the top sheet of plastic, invert the pastry into the pan, and mold to fit. Remove the plastic and trim the edges. Prick the dough with a fork. Bake for 16 to 18 minutes, or until golden brown.

4. In a medium saucepan, whisk together the milk, egg, cornstarch, the remaining ½ cup sugar, and the remaining ⅛ teaspoon salt. Whisking constantly, bring to a boil over medium heat, then lower the heat. Whisk for 30 seconds or until thickened and smooth. Gradually whisk in the half-and-half and cook for 1 minute. Remove from the heat and stir in the vanilla. Pour the filling into the warm shell, cover it with the plastic touching the surface, and chill for 2 hours or overnight.

5. Just before serving, arrange the apricots, kiwifruit, and raspberries in a decorative pattern on top.

Makes 8 servings

Per serving: 287 calories, 10 g fat, 28 mg cholesterol, 2 g fiber, 185 mg sodium

Tropical Fruit Trifle Parfaits

Invite the refreshing taste of the islands to your party.

    1 pint mango sorbet
    1 cup diced fresh pineapple (see note)
   12 gingersnaps
    2 containers (6 ounces each) low-fat piña colada yogurt

1. Place ½ cup of the sorbet in each of 4 tall parfait glasses. Top with half of the pineapple.

2. Crumble 2 gingersnaps into each glass. Spoon 2 tablespoons yogurt into each glass. Add the remaining sorbet, pineapple, and yogurt in layers. Stand 1 gingersnap vertically in each glass.

Makes 4 servings

Per serving: 247 calories, 8 g fat, 3 mg cholesterol, 1 g fiber, 134 mg sodium

Note: If you don't have fresh pineapple, substitute 1 can (8 ounces) crushed pineapple, drained.

HEALTHY HORS D'OEUVRES IN A HURRY

Hors d'oeuvres may be small, but they can present big problems for even the most health conscious among us. Use the list below to make a quick sweep through your supermarket, then whip up small but mighty taste sensations.

From the Freezer Case

FROZEN TORTELLINI. Cook tortellini according to package directions. Let cool. Spear one or two tortellini onto a skewer. Fan out the skewers on a serving tray or place them upright in a vase. Serve with any of these dipping sauces:

■ Prepared pesto

■ Light or fat-free mayonnaise blended with Dijon mustard and a few drops of lemon juice

■ Red pepper sauce: Drain a jar of roasted red peppers, season with fresh or dried herbs (or roasted garlic), salt to taste, and puree in a blender until chunky/smooth.

FROZEN MINI-PIEROGIES. Bake mini-pierogies according to package directions. When cool enough to handle, spear onto skewers and arrange on a serving tray. For a choice of dipping sauces, offer the following:

■ Prepared salsa blended with fat-free plain yogurt and chopped fresh cilantro

■ 1 tablespoon prepared horseradish mixed with 1 cup light sour cream, 1 teaspoon caraway seeds, and a few drops of lemon juice

■ Onion-bacon dip: Cook 3 or 4 strips of turkey bacon until crisp. Drain, cool, and crumble. Coat a skillet with cooking spray and add 1 chopped large onion. Cook, stirring, for 5 minutes or until tender. Let cool. Mix bacon and onion with ½ cup light sour cream, 2 tablespoons light or fat-free mayonnaise, and freshly ground black pepper.

From the Deli Counter

SMOKED SALMON. Puree sliced smoked salmon in a blender with a few drops of lemon juice until smooth. Now, get creative with the salmon pâté.

■ Spread the salmon pâté on thin, toasted baguette slices. Top with finely chopped scallions or paper-thin slices of peeled, seeded cucumber and freshly ground pepper.

■ Select perfect arugula leaves. Wash and dry them thoroughly. Spoon the pâté onto the bottom halves of the leaves. Sprinkle with capers and chopped chives. Roll up the leaves and secure with wooden picks.

■ Drain canned hearts of palm. Dry thoroughly. Cut crosswise into medium rounds. Spread each with the pâté, then sprinkle with crumbled blue cheese.

PRECOOKED SHRIMP. Use easy precooked shrimp as the centerpiece of one of these taste-tempting creations.

■ Fill baked mini-phyllo pastry shells (look for the prebaked variety*) with a spoonful of softened herb cheese, such as Boursin. Nestle a small shrimp on top and sprinkle with chopped fresh parsley or chives.

■ Place spoonfuls of prepared taramasalata (look for jars of this Greek spread in the dairy case) into the cupped ends of washed and dried endive leaves. Top each with a shrimp. Sprinkle with chopped fresh dill.

SMOKED HAM OR TURKEY. Ask the counterperson to cut thin, uniform slices. Coat one side of each slice with any of the following spreads, then roll them up and secure them with wooden picks.

■ Blended light cream cheese and prepared chutney

■ Blended grainy mustard and chopped cornichons (tiny French sour pickles available in jars) or finely chopped half-sour pickles

■ Blended blue cheese, chopped dates, and chopped pecans

From the Grocery

Keep these versatile ingredients in your pantry. Besides mixing and matching well with many of the suggestions above, they'll help inspire you to create winning combinations of your own.

CANNED CHICKPEAS. Puree in a blender along with some garlic, cumin, or prepared salsa to taste. Use as a dip for baked tortilla chips or toasted pita wedges.

PREPARED TAPENADE. This Provençal olive spread, available in jars, is an ideal dip or filling on its own.

ANCHOVY PASTE. Available in tubes, it's perfect for combining with any low-fat, creamy-style cheese and spooning into hollowed cherry tomatoes.

ARTICHOKE HEARTS. The ones that are packed in water, not oil, can be tossed with low-fat dressing and added to skewers along with other bite-size foods such as mini-shrimp, roasted red peppers, and cherry tomatoes.

*To order mini-pastry shells and other phyllo products, call (800) OK-FILLO (653-4556) or visit the Web site www.fillofactory.com.

Having a healthy holiday doesn't mean depriving yourself of great food. To prove it, we've put together a Thanksgiving feast that you and your family will love. Indulge in roast turkey, cranberry sauce, green beans, and candied sweet potatoes.

Roasted Turkey Breast with Cranberry Sauce

Here's a clever way to reduce the fat in your holiday bird. Use only the lean, tasty breast and marinate it overnight in a flavorful mixture of crushed spices and yogurt.

Cranberry Sauce

2	cups fresh cranberries
½	cup dried apple slices
	Grated peel of 1 orange
1	cup orange juice
½	cup all-fruit apple butter
3	tablespoons maple syrup

Turkey

1	boneless, skinless turkey breast half (about 2¼ pounds)
¾	cup fat-free plain yogurt
2	cloves garlic, finely chopped
1	tablespoon apple cider vinegar
1	teaspoon black peppercorns, crushed
1	teaspoon cumin seed, crushed
1	teaspoon dried rosemary, crushed
1	teaspoon finely chopped fresh ginger
½	teaspoon ground cinnamon

1. *To make the cranberry sauce:* In a food processor or blender, combine the cranberries, apples, orange peel, and orange juice. Pulse until finely chopped but not pureed. Transfer to a medium saucepan. Add the apple butter and maple syrup. Bring to a boil over high heat. Reduce the heat to low and simmer, uncovered, for 10 minutes. Transfer to a serving bowl and allow to cool. Cover and refrigerate.

2. *To make the turkey:* Rinse the turkey with cold water and pat dry with paper towels. Set aside.

3. In a large glass or stainless steel mixing bowl, combine the yogurt, garlic, vinegar, pepper, cumin, rosemary, ginger, and cinnamon. Add the turkey and turn to coat evenly. Cover and refrigerate overnight, turning the meat occasionally.

4. To roast the turkey, remove it from the marinade and place it in an oven cooking bag. Discard the marinade. Roast according to the package directions or until the internal temperature of the turkey reaches 170°F. Start checking the internal temperature after 1 hour.

5. Remove the turkey from the cooking bag and let stand for 10 minutes before slicing and serving. Serve with the cranberry sauce.

Makes 8 servings

Per serving: 252 calories, 1.5 g fat, 85 mg cholesterol, 2 g fiber, 76 mg sodium

Ginger Green Beans

These fragrant green beans are ready in less than 15 minutes.

　1　**package (16 ounces) frozen whole green beans**
　1　**tablespoon trans-free tub-style margarine**
　½　**cup chopped shallots**
　1　**tablespoon chopped crystallized ginger**
　½　**teaspoon grated lemon peel**
　⅛　**teaspoon freshly ground black pepper**

1. In a medium saucepan, bring 1" of water to a boil. Place the beans on a steaming rack and set the rack in the pan. Cover and steam for 7 to 9 minutes, or until tender. Remove the steaming rack and set aside. Drain the pan.

2. In the same pan, melt the margarine over low heat. Add the shallots and ginger. Cook for 4 minutes, or until the shallots are tender. Add the beans, lemon peel, and pepper. Cook for 1 minute, or until heated through.

Makes 8 servings

Per serving: 39 calories, 1.5 g fat, 0 mg cholesterol, 1 g fiber, 28 mg sodium

Candied Sweet Potatoes

This holiday favorite can be included in a healthy menu. We kept in just enough of the "candy" so it tastes delicious but isn't overloaded with excess fat and sugar.

1¼   **pounds sweet potatoes, peeled and cut into 2" pieces**
½   **cup chopped onion**
1   **Granny Smith apple, cut into 1" pieces**
¼   **cup raisins**
¼   **cup orange juice**
2   **tablespoons brown sugar**
2   **tablespoons trans-free tub-style margarine**
½   **teaspoon grated orange peel**

1. In a large saucepan, combine the sweet potatoes and onion. Add 1" of water to the pan. Cover and simmer over medium heat for 10 minutes, or until the sweet potatoes are tender. Drain and return the vegetables to the pan.

2. Add the apple, raisins, orange juice, brown sugar, margarine, and orange peel. Cook over low heat, stirring frequently, until the liquid reduces slightly and glazes the sweet potatoes and apples.

Makes 8 servings

Per serving: 127 calories, 3 g fat, 0 mg cholesterol, 1 g fiber, 48 mg sodium

Every year at Christmas, many of us serve the same old fatty roast beef, turkey, or ham, with sugary cakes and pies for dessert. This year, make something special. Give your family a Christmas dinner that has all the holiday trimmings with just a fraction of the fat. The centerpiece of this meal is a savory roast pork tenderloin.

Hot Mulled Apple-Cranberry Punch

Looking for a little Christmas spirit? This warm beverage is spiced just right to put you and your guests in the holiday mood.

4	cups water
3	cups fresh or frozen cranberries (see note)
3	cups apple cider
½	cup sugar
1	cinnamon stick, broken into pieces
1	teaspoon whole cloves
⅛	teaspoon ground nutmeg
	Peel of 1 orange, cut in 1 continuous strip
	Cinnamon sticks and orange slices

1. In a large saucepan, combine the water, cranberries, cider, sugar, cinnamon stick, cloves, nutmeg, and orange peel. Bring to a boil over medium-high heat. When the cranberries begin to pop, reduce the heat to low. Cover and simmer for 10 to 15 minutes, or until the berries are tender.

2. Strain the mixture, discarding the solids. Pour into mugs and serve warm garnished with the cinnamon sticks and orange slices.

Makes 6 cups

Per ¾ cup: 118 calories, 0 g fat, 0 mg cholesterol, 2 g fiber, 3 mg sodium

Note: If cranberries are unavailable, you can replace the cranberries, water, and sugar with 3 cups cranberry juice cocktail.

Variations

■ Hot Mulled Cranberry-Apricot Punch: Replace the apple cider with apricot nectar.

■ Hot Mulled Cranberry-Pear Punch: Replace the apple cider with pear nectar.

Glazed Roast Pork Tenderloin

Here's a surefire hit for the holidays. Juicy roast pork tenderloin is glazed with an irresistible mixture of honey, mustard, orange, and cinnamon. And it takes only 30 minutes to cook.

- ¼ cup Dijon mustard
- 2 tablespoons orange juice
- 2 tablespoons honey
- 1 teaspoon grated orange peel
- ¼ teaspoon ground cinnamon
- ⅛ teaspoon ground allspice
- 2 pounds pork tenderloin, trimmed of all visible fat

1. Preheat the oven to 325°F.
2. In a small bowl, whisk together the mustard, orange juice, honey, orange peel, cinnamon, and allspice.
3. Place the pork on a rack in a shallow roasting pan. Insert a meat thermometer into the center of the pork. Roast for 30 minutes, or until the thermometer registers 160°F. During the last 10 minutes of roasting, brush the pork occasionally with the mustard mixture.
4. Remove from the oven and let stand for 5 minutes before slicing.

Makes 8 servings

Per serving: 162 calories, 4.5 g fat, 65 mg cholesterol, 0 g fiber, 147 mg sodium

Herbed Peas and Onions

Thyme, dill, and sautéed onions give sweet peas a savory flavor that pairs well with almost any main dish.

- 1 tablespoon extra-virgin olive oil
- 2 onions, thinly sliced and separated into rings
- 1 cup fat-free, reduced-sodium chicken broth
- 2 teaspoons dried thyme
- 1 teaspoon salt-free lemon-herb seasoning
- 2 packages (10 ounces each) frozen peas, thawed
- 2 tablespoons chopped fresh dill

1. Warm the oil in a large skillet over medium heat. Add the onions and cook, stirring frequently, for 6 to 8 minutes, or until lightly browned.

2. Stir in the broth, thyme, and lemon-herb seasoning. Bring to a boil over high heat. Reduce the heat to low and stir in the peas. Cover and cook for 6 to 8 minutes, or until the peas are heated through. Uncover and cook for 1 minute, or until most of the liquid evaporates. Sprinkle with the dill.

Makes 8 servings

Per serving: 89 calories, 2 g fat, 0 mg cholesterol, 3 g fiber, 71 mg sodium

HOLIDAY DRESS-UPS

Angel food cake is about as light a cake as you can hope for. Made from egg whites, it's fat-free and lower in calories than most other cakes. It's an ideal way to end a big holiday meal. You can serve it plain, dusted with confectioners' sugar, or adorned with fresh fruit. Or turn it into something extraordinary with these suggestions.

■ Dip fresh or dried fruit (such as strawberries, whole cherries, or apricots) into melted chocolate. Allow to dry and arrange the fruit on top of the cake.

■ Pour melted chocolate into a small, resealable plastic bag and snip off one tiny corner. Draw on top of the cake in a decorative design.

■ Make a quick strawberry or raspberry sauce: In a food processor, puree 2 cups unsweetened frozen strawberries or raspberries (thawed), 2 tablespoons sugar, and 1 tablespoon lemon juice. This keeps in the refrigerator for up to 2 days.

■ Mix grated orange peel into slightly softened, frozen low-fat vanilla or chocolate yogurt and serve alongside cake slices.

The Passover seder meal commemorates Jewish heritage with a variety of symbolic foods. We've updated these dishes to cut fat, calories, and cholesterol without sacrificing flavor.

Charoset

Charoset is a simple fruit-and-nut mixture that represents the mortar and bricks that the captive Israelites used to build the cities of Egypt. This version has less fat and sugar than traditional recipes and still tastes delicious.

- 1   Red Delicious apple, finely chopped
- ¼   cup finely chopped toasted walnuts (see note)
- ¼   cup chopped dates
- ¼   cup dark raisins
- 2   tablespoons sweet red wine or grape juice
- 1   tablespoon sugar
- ¼   teaspoon ground cinnamon

1. In a medium bowl, stir together the apple, walnuts, dates, raisins, wine or grape juice, sugar, and cinnamon. Refrigerate for 10 minutes before serving.

Makes about 2 cups

Per ¼ cup: 72 calories, 2.5 g fat, 0 mg cholesterol, 1 g fiber, 3 mg sodium

Note: To toast the walnuts, place them in a dry nonstick skillet over medium heat and shake the skillet often for 3 to 5 minutes, or until the nuts are fragrant.

Passover Spinach Squares

Serve these as an appetizer with the main course. You can replace the fresh spinach with 3 packages (10 ounces each) thawed frozen chopped spinach.

1½	pounds fresh spinach, stemmed and washed
1½	teaspoons canola oil
1	leek, thinly sliced (white part only)
2	cloves garlic, finely chopped
2	teaspoons lemon juice
¾	teaspoon dried oregano
⅛	teaspoon freshly ground black pepper
3	egg whites

1. Preheat the oven to 350°F. Coat an 8" × 8" baking dish with cooking spray.

2. Bring a small amount of water to a boil in a large pot over medium heat. Add the spinach, cover, and cook for 5 minutes, or until the spinach is wilted. Squeeze the spinach dry, chop, and place in a large bowl.

3. Warm the oil in a small skillet over low heat. Add the leek and garlic. Cook, stirring often, for 10 minutes, or until tender but not browned. Add to the spinach. Stir in the lemon juice, oregano, and pepper.

4. Place the egg whites in a medium bowl. Beat until foamy using an electric mixer. Gently stir into the spinach mixture. Pour it into the prepared pan and bake for 35 minutes, or until set. Let cool slightly before cutting. Serve warm.

Makes 16 servings

Per serving: 22 calories, 1 g fat, 0 mg cholesterol, 1 g fiber, 45 mg sodium

Easter dinner provides the perfect opportunity to showcase the bounty of spring in one special meal. This menu includes carrots, spring greens with strawberries, and an extraordinary roast lamb loin.

Spring Greens and Strawberries with Poppy Seed Dressing

Tangy watercress and arugula get a touch of sweetness from orange juice, poppy seeds, and strawberries.

3 cups watercress leaves
3 cups torn arugula leaves
3 cups sliced strawberries
¼ cup orange juice
2 teaspoons olive oil
2 teaspoons poppy seeds
½ teaspoon grated orange peel

1. In a large bowl, mix the watercress, arugula, and strawberries.
2. In a small bowl, whisk together the orange juice, oil, poppy seeds, and orange peel. Pour over the salad and toss gently to combine.

Makes 8 servings

Per serving: 37 calories, 2 g fat, 0 mg cholesterol, 1 g fiber, 8 mg sodium

Spicy Lamb Loin

Tender lamb loin is served over orzo and topped with a simple sauce featuring thyme, shallots, and balsamic vinegar. The whole dish comes together in less than 45 minutes.

2	pounds boneless lamb loin, trimmed of all visible fat
2	tablespoons black peppercorns, crushed
2	tablespoons coriander seeds, crushed
½	cup balsamic vinegar
2	tablespoons finely chopped shallots
1	teaspoon dried thyme
2	bay leaves
2	cups fat-free, reduced-sodium beef broth
4	teaspoons butter or trans-free margarine
¼	cup finely chopped parsley
6	cups cooked orzo

1. Preheat the oven to 400°F.

2. Cut the lamb loin into 4 fillets. Firmly press the peppercorns and coriander into both sides of each fillet.

3. Coat a large nonstick skillet with cooking spray and warm over medium-high heat. Sear the fillets on both sides, then transfer to an ovenproof pan. Roast for 10 to 15 minutes. Remove from the oven and set aside for 5 minutes.

4. Return the skillet to medium heat. Add the vinegar, shallots, thyme, and bay leaves. Cook for 3 to 4 minutes, scraping any browned bits from the bottom of the skillet. Stir in the broth and bring to a boil. Boil for 2 to 3 minutes, or until the liquid is slightly reduced.

5. Reduce the heat to low and whisk in the butter or margarine. Stir in the parsley. Remove and discard the bay leaves. Keep the mixture warm.

6. Cut the lamb into very thin slices. Serve with the orzo and drizzle the sauce over the lamb.

Makes 8 servings

Per serving: 380 calories, 11 g fat, 79 mg cholesterol, 0 g fiber, 97 mg sodium

Candied Carrot Coins

The sweet flavor of candied carrots is welcome in any menu. Plus, they're packed with health-boosting beta-carotene.

  2   **pounds carrots, sliced ¼" thick**

  1   **cup brown sugar**

  1   **tablespoon trans-free tub-style margarine**

1. Bring 2" of water to a boil in a medium saucepan. Place the carrots on a steaming rack and set the rack in the pan. Cover and steam for 15 minutes, or until tender. Remove the steaming rack and set aside.

2. Measure 1 cup of the cooking liquid and discard the remainder. Return the liquid to the pan and add the brown sugar and margarine. Bring to a boil over high heat. Stir until the sugar dissolves. Reduce the heat to low and simmer for 10 minutes, or until the liquid reduces slightly. Add the carrots and cook for 10 minutes, or until the liquid is reduced and the carrots are glazed.

Makes 6 servings

Per serving: 221 calories, 2 g fat, 0 mg cholesterol, 5 g fiber, 138 mg sodium

Your family won't eat healthy fare, and you can't resist their goodies.

What you need: healthy home-style recipes

It's difficult for a family raised on sloppy joes and fries to suddenly see their plates filled with grilled chicken and broccoli. And let's face it: It's not so easy on you either. These recipes—which include pot roast, lasagna, and baked potatoes—can ease the transition: They're both healthy and hearty. And your family will love them.

COMMONSENSE STRATEGY:
Get into the habit of buying *colorful* vegetables—deep-purple eggplant, emerald-green Swiss chard, jewel-toned red and orange peppers, sunset-hued sweet potatoes. The deeper the color, the denser the nutrients.

Whole Wheat Pancakes

These pancakes are so easy you needn't reserve them for just weekends.

1¼	cups whole wheat flour	⅛	teaspoon salt
¼	cup toasted wheat germ	1½	cups fat-free milk
1½	teaspoons baking powder	¼	cup fat-free liquid egg substitute
½	teaspoon ground cinnamon	1	tablespoon butter, melted

1. In a large bowl, mix the flour, wheat germ, baking powder, cinnamon, and salt. Add the milk, egg substitute, and butter. Mix just until the ingredients are blended. Do not overbeat.

2. Coat a large nonstick skillet with cooking spray. Warm over medium-high heat until a drop of water sizzles when dropped into the skillet. Using a ¼-cup measuring cup as a ladle, scoop out slightly less than ¼ cup of batter for each pancake. Drop the batter into the pan, being careful not to crowd the pancakes.

3. Cook for 2 minutes or until the edges begin to look dry. Turn and cook for 1 minute, or until browned on the bottom. Remove from the pan.

4. Take the skillet off the heat and coat with more cooking spray. Continue until all the batter is used.

Makes 12

Per 3 pancakes: 221 calories, 4.5 g fat, 10 mg cholesterol, 6 g fiber, 325 mg sodium

Note: Place the pancakes on a baking sheet in a 175°F oven to keep them warm until all are cooked. Serve with maple syrup or honey.

QUICK AND HEALTHY RECIPES FOR THE 10 MOST TREACHEROUS DANGER ZONES

Chicken and Black Bean Lasagna

To easily freeze lasagna, line the baking dish with foil before assembling the lasagna; freeze uncovered. When frozen, remove the lasagna from the dish, wrap in the foil, and return to the freezer.

1	can (28 ounces) tomatoes, drained and chopped
1	can (4 ounces) chopped green chile peppers, drained
1	can (8 ounces) low-sodium tomato sauce
1	can (15 ounces) black beans, rinsed and drained
1	teaspoon ground cumin
1	teaspoon chili powder
6	no-boil lasagna noodles
1½	cups fat-free ricotta cheese
2	cups chopped cooked chicken breast
2	cups shredded reduced-fat Cheddar cheese

1. Preheat the oven to 375°F. Coat an 8" × 8" baking dish with cooking spray.

2. In a medium bowl, mix the tomatoes, peppers, and tomato sauce. In a small bowl, mix the beans, cumin, and chili powder. Lightly mash the beans with a fork.

3. Spoon ½ cup of the tomato mixture into the prepared baking dish. Place 2 of the noodles over the sauce. Top with one-third of the beans, one-third of the ricotta cheese, and one-third of the chicken. Cover with ½ cup of the Cheddar cheese and one-third of the remaining tomato sauce.

4. Repeat twice. Top with the remaining ½ cup Cheddar cheese. Bake for 30 minutes, or until bubbling.

Makes 4 servings

Per serving: 347 calories, 9 g fat, 51 mg cholesterol, 7 g fiber, 738 mg sodium

Old-Fashioned Pot Roast

Roasts usually are not sold in the 1-pound piece called for here, so have the butcher cut off that much and freeze the remainder to use at another time.

1	beef top round roast (1½ pounds), trimmed of all visible fat
1	cup tomato juice
½	cup red wine or fat-free beef broth
1	tablespoon Dijon mustard
1	teaspoon dried rosemary
1	pound baby carrots
¾	pound small red potatoes, peeled
8	small onions
3	ribs celery, sliced into 1" pieces

1. Preheat the oven to 325°F.

2. Coat an ovenproof Dutch oven with cooking spray. Add the beef and brown on all sides over medium-high heat. Transfer to a plate. Add the tomato juice, wine or broth, mustard, and rosemary to the pot. Mix well and bring to a boil over high heat. Return the beef to the pot.

3. Cover and bake for 45 minutes. Add the carrots, potatoes, onions, and celery. Cover and bake for 45 to 60 minutes, or until the beef is tender.

Makes 6 servings

Per serving: 334 calories, 11 g fat, 56 mg cholesterol, 5 g fiber, 289 mg sodium

Sautéed Steak and Mushrooms

Crimini mushrooms add extra rich flavor but no fat to this dish. The healthy way to eat meat is to pair lean cuts with lots of veggies.

1 pound sirloin steak
¼ teaspoon salt
⅛ teaspoon freshly ground black pepper
1 package (6–8 ounces) sliced crimini mushrooms
¼ cup water
1 teaspoon Worcestershire sauce
½ teaspoon finely chopped garlic

1. Coat a large skillet with cooking spray and place over medium-high heat. Sprinkle the steak with the salt and pepper. Add to the pan and cook for 6 to 7 minutes. Mist the steak with the cooking spray, turn, and cook for 6 to 7 minutes longer for medium-rare. Transfer to a plate, cover, and keep warm.

2. Add the mushrooms, water, Worcestershire sauce, and garlic to the skillet. Stir to scrape up any brown bits. Cook for 5 minutes, or until the mushrooms soften. Slice the steak and top with the cooked mushrooms.

Makes 4 servings

Per serving: 205 calories, 14 g fat, 57 mg cholesterol, 1 g fiber, 193 mg sodium

Whipped Carrots and Potatoes

Here's a three-in-one vegetable dish that'll have 'em guessing what's in it.

3	medium carrots, sliced
1	small potato, peeled and sliced
1	small onion, chopped
1	tablespoon fat-free milk
1	teaspoon reduced-calorie trans-free margarine
¼	teaspoon dried tarragon
⅛	teaspoon freshly ground black pepper

1. Place the carrots, potato, and onion in a medium saucepan and add enough water to cover. Bring to a boil over high heat, then reduce the heat to medium-low. Cover and simmer for 25 minutes, or until the vegetables are very tender. Drain and transfer to a medium bowl.

2. Using an electric mixer or a potato masher, mash the vegetables. Mix in the milk, margarine, tarragon, and pepper.

Makes 4 servings

Per serving: 70 calories, 1 g fat, 0 mg cholesterol, 3 g fiber, 35 mg sodium

Zucchini in Fresh Tomato Sauce

Whether you grow your own zucchini and tomatoes or pick them up at the farmers' market, here's a low-fat way to savor these summer staples.

1	small onion, thinly sliced
2	medium tomatoes, chopped
1	tablespoon finely chopped parsley
½	teaspoon dried oregano
¼	teaspoon dried marjoram
⅛	teaspoon cracked black pepper
1½	cups zucchini sliced ¼" thick
2	tablespoons shredded reduced-fat mozzarella cheese

1. Coat a large skillet with cooking spray and warm over medium heat. Add the onion and cook for 4 minutes. Stir in the tomatoes, parsley, oregano, marjoram, and pepper. Cook for 2 minutes, or until heated through.

2. Stir in the zucchini. Cover and cook for 4 to 5 minutes, or until the zucchini is crisp-tender. Sprinkle with the cheese.

Makes 4 servings

Per serving: 50 calories, 1.5 g fat, 4 mg cholesterol, 2 g fiber, 41 mg sodium

Baked Potatoes with Chive and Cheese Topping

So who needs butter on a baked potato when there's a creamy low-fat topping like this one around?

4	medium baking potatoes
¼	cup fat-free cottage cheese
2	tablespoons finely chopped chives
2	tablespoons fat-free plain yogurt
1	tablespoon grated Parmesan cheese
⅛	teaspoon dried basil

1. Preheat the oven to 400°F.

2. Scrub the potatoes with cold water, then pat dry. Use a fork to prick the potatoes in several places. Place on a baking sheet and bake for 40 to 60 minutes, or until tender.

3. In a blender, process the cottage cheese, chives, yogurt, Parmesan cheese, and basil until smooth.

4. Cut an X in the top of each potato. Push in the ends and use a fork to lightly fluff the pulp. Spoon the cheese mixture over the potatoes.

Makes 4 servings

Per serving: 127 calories, 1 g fat, 2 mg cholesterol, 3 g fiber, 71 mg sodium

Serendipitous Spinach Salad

When you're looking for a new salad idea, try this change of pace—apples and grapes tossed with spinach and topped with a creamy honey-lime dressing. For variety, substitute peaches and kiwifruit for the other fruit.

4	**cups torn spinach**
1	**medium apple or pear, coarsely chopped**
¼	**cup seedless red grapes, halved**
¼	**cup sliced celery**
¼	**cup fat-free plain yogurt**
1	**tablespoon honey**
¼	**teaspoon grated lime peel**

1. In a large bowl, mix the spinach, apple or pear, grapes, and celery.

2. In a small bowl, mix the yogurt, honey, and lime peel. Drizzle over the spinach mixture. Gently toss until lightly coated.

Makes 4 servings

Per serving: 62 calories, 0.5 g fat, 0 mg cholesterol, 2 g fiber, 62 mg sodium

Cranberry-Apple Cobbler

Nobody will refuse this yummy sweet—and they'll never guess how good it is for them. For an extra special treat, top with fat-free frozen vanilla yogurt or ice cream.

¾ cup fresh or frozen cranberries

2½ cups sliced tart apples

2 tablespoons + ½ teaspoon sugar

¼ teaspoon + ⅛ teaspoon ground cinnamon

½ cup reduced-fat biscuit mix

⅔ cup buttermilk

½ teaspoon grated orange peel

Pinch of nutmeg

1. Preheat the oven to 375°F. Coat an 8" × 8" baking dish with cooking spray.

2. In a medium bowl, mix the cranberries, apples, 2 tablespoons of the sugar, and ¼ teaspoon of the cinnamon. Spoon into the prepared baking dish. Bake for 20 minutes or until the fruit is almost tender.

3. In a small bowl, mix the biscuit mix, buttermilk, orange peel, and nutmeg. Spoon over fruit mixture. Mix the remaining ½ teaspoon sugar with the remaining ⅛ teaspoon cinnamon and sprinkle over the biscuit topping.

4. Bake for 15 minutes or until the biscuits are golden brown.

Makes 4 servings

Per serving: 141 calories, 1 g fat, 1 mg cholesterol, 2 g fiber, 216 mg sodium

Sunset Compote

If you can't live on a tropical island, here's a dessert that will at least make you feel as if you're on one.

1	medium papaya, peeled and cubed
2	kiwifruits, peeled and sliced
4	cups strawberries, quartered
2	tablespoons lime juice
¼	teaspoon almond extract
2	tablespoons toasted and chopped pistachios

1. In a medium bowl, mix the papaya, kiwifruit, and strawberries. Drizzle with the lime juice and almond extract. Gently toss until coated. Serve sprinkled with the pistachios.

Makes 6 servings

Per serving: 82 calories, 2 g fat, 0 mg cholesterol, 4 g fiber, 4 mg sodium

From November 1 to March 31, your willpower goes south with the geese.

What you need: savory cold-weather eats

When the wind blows cold and you're continually chilled to the bone, cooking and eating in a warm, cozy kitchen can be a comfort. It's even more comforting to know that these stick-to-your-ribs meals won't stick to the rest of you—all are made with low-fat, healthy ingredients.

COMMONSENSE STRATEGY: When the temperature drops, it's natural to crave creamy, stick-to-your-ribs favorites. But don't let your urge to cozy up to high-fat, high-calorie foods let you ignore your veggies. You'll find several tempting vegetable dishes below.

Easiest Chili Ever

You probably have most of these ingredients in the house already.

- 1 tablespoon olive oil
- 1–2 tablespoons chili powder
- 1 tablespoon dehydrated onion
- 1 can (28 ounces) whole tomatoes
- 1 can (14–16 ounces) Italian-style stewed tomatoes
- 1 can (14 ounces) chili beans
- ½ package (12 ounces) soy crumbles (such as Green Giant Harvest Burgers for Recipes)

1. Warm the oil in a large saucepan over medium heat. Stir in the chili powder and onion. Cook for 30 seconds. Add the whole tomatoes, stewed tomatoes, beans, and soy crumbles. Break up the whole tomatoes with a wooden spoon. Cook for 20 minutes, or until heated through.

Makes 4 servings

Per serving: 244 calories, 7 g fat, 0 mg cholesterol, 9 g fiber, 1,304 mg sodium

Note: This recipe was created by Diana Dyer.

Spicy Lentils

*Cooking time for lentils can vary from 15 minutes to as long
as 1 hour, depending on the type and age of the lentils. Red lentils
(which turn yellow when cooked) cook very quickly because they are split,
and after 15 to 20 minutes, they soften to a puree. Brown lentils hold
their shape better but can take longer to cook. Serve this stewlike
dish in a shallow bowl over brown rice.*

1 tablespoon canola oil

1 cup finely chopped onion

2 teaspoons ground ginger

1 teaspoon ground cumin

1 cup dried red or brown lentils

3 cups water

¾ teaspoon salt

2 tablespoons finely chopped fresh cilantro

1 tablespoon lemon juice

1. Warm the oil in a medium saucepan over medium heat. Add the onion
and cook, stirring often, for 5 minutes, or until tender. Stir in the ginger
and cumin and cook for 30 seconds.

2. Add the lentils, water, and salt. Bring to a boil. Reduce the heat to low
and simmer, partially covered, for 15 minutes. If the lentils are soft, uncover and gently boil until most of the liquid evaporates. If the lentils are
not yet tender, continue to cook, partially covered, testing every 10 minutes or so.

3. Stir in the cilantro and lemon juice.

Makes 4 servings

Per serving: 167 calories, 4 g fat, 0 mg cholesterol, 6 g fiber, 406 mg sodium

Bouillabaisse

This traditional French stew brimming with seafood is ideal for wintry evenings. Serve in crockery bowls with crunchy toast and a tossed salad.

    1   tablespoon olive oil
    2   bottles (8 ounces each) clam juice
    1   cup chopped onion
    2   leeks, thinly sliced
    5   cloves garlic, finely chopped
    ¾   pound small red potatoes, quartered
    1   can (28 ounces) chopped Italian plum tomatoes (with juice)
    1   pound halibut, cut into 2" cubes
    ½   pound bay scallops
    ½   pound large shrimp, peeled and deveined
    2–3 tablespoons chopped fresh tarragon or basil
        Salt
        Freshly ground black pepper

1. Bring the oil and ¼ cup of the clam juice to a boil in a soup pot over medium-high heat. Add the onion, leeks, garlic, and potatoes. Cook for 5 minutes, or until the onions are lightly browned. Add the tomatoes (with juice). Bring to a boil. Cook for 10 minutes.

2. Add the halibut, scallops, and shrimp. Cook for 5 minutes, or until the fish flakes easily when tested with a fork. Stir in the tarragon or basil. Season with the salt and pepper.

Makes 4 servings

Per serving: 420 calories, 8 g fat, 148 mg cholesterol, 3 g fiber, 474 mg sodium

Cioppino

Created years ago by San Francisco's Italian immigrants, cioppino (chuh-PEE-noh) is a rich tomato stew chock-full of seafood. This low-fat version features shrimp, clams, and haddock. For real Frisco flair, serve it with sourdough bread. (See recipe on page 306.)

1	small onion, chopped
4	scallions, sliced
2	cloves garlic, finely chopped
1½	cups fat-free, reduced-sodium chicken broth
2	canned plum tomatoes (with juice), chopped
¼	cup finely chopped parsley
1	bay leaf
⅛	teaspoon dried thyme
	Pinch of dried rosemary
	Pinch of ground red pepper
	Pinch of freshly ground black pepper
½	pound medium shrimp, peeled and deveined
8	littleneck clams, scrubbed
½	pound haddock fillets, cut into 1½" pieces

1. Coat a large saucepan with cooking spray and place over medium heat. Add the onion, scallions, and garlic. Cook over medium heat for 3 minutes.

2. Add broth, tomatoes (with juice), parsley, bay leaf, thyme, rosemary, red pepper, and black pepper. Cover and bring to a boil. Reduce the heat. Simmer for 30 minutes.

3. Add the shrimp, clams, and haddock. Cover and bring just to a boil, then reduce the heat. Gently simmer for 5 minutes, or until the shrimp turn pink, the clams open, and the fish flakes easily when tested with a fork. Remove and discard the bay leaf and any unopened clams.

Makes 4 servings

Per serving: 238 calories, 3.5 g fat, 158 mg cholesterol, 1 g fiber, 318 mg sodium

Pork and Vegetable Stew with Cornmeal Dumplings

Dumplings ordinarily add unwanted fat to stews, but these fluffy cornmeal dumplings contain only a small amount of oil.

Stew

¾ pound lean boneless pork, trimmed of all visible fat

2 teaspoons canola oil

2 medium onions, cut into thin wedges

1 clove garlic, finely chopped

4 cups fat-free beef broth

1 teaspoon dried marjoram

½ teaspoon dried thyme

¼ teaspoon freshly ground black pepper

2 cups peeled and cubed sweet potatoes

2 cups frozen peas

3 tablespoons all-purpose flour

3 tablespoons cold water

Dumplings

¼ cup all-purpose flour

¼ cup cornmeal

1 tablespoon finely chopped parsley

¾ teaspoon baking powder

⅛ teaspoon dried marjoram

3 tablespoons fat-free milk

1 tablespoon canola oil

1. *To make the stew:* Cut the pork into 1" pieces. Coat a 4-quart Dutch oven with cooking spray. Add the oil and swirl to coat the bottom. Warm over medium-high heat. Add the pork, onions, and garlic. Stir until the meat is browned.

2. Stir in the broth, marjoram, thyme, and pepper. Cover and bring to a boil over high heat, then reduce the heat to medium. Simmer for 30 minutes, or until the meat is almost tender.

3. Stir in the sweet potatoes. Cover and simmer for 20 minutes. Stir in the peas. Cover and simmer for 5 minutes, or until the vegetables are just tender.

4. In a small bowl, mix the flour and water. Stir into the pork mixture. Stir until the mixture thickens and begins to gently boil.

5. *To make the dumplings:* In a small bowl, mix the flour, cornmeal, parsley, baking powder, and marjoram. In another small bowl, mix the milk and oil. Pour over the flour mixture and stir with a fork just until all the flour is moistened.

6. Spoon the cornmeal mixture into five mounds on top of the stew. Reduce the heat to medium-low, cover, and simmer for 10 to 12 minutes, or until the dumplings are no longer doughy in the center.

Makes 5 servings

Per serving: 412 calories, 11.5 g fat, 38 mg cholesterol, 7 g fiber, 203 mg sodium

Note: To check the doneness of the dumplings, carefully poke a wooden pick into the center of one. If no dough clings to the wooden pick, the dumplings are done. If some dough clings, cover the pot and cook the dumplings for 1 or 2 minutes longer. Then check again with a clean wooden pick.

Turkey Divan with Peaches

Here's a divine dish! And it's all the more so because it's minus the heavy cream sauce and egg yolks that characterize classic turkey divan.

> 2 turkey breast tenderloins (about 1 pound total)
> 1 package (16 ounces) frozen cut broccoli
> ½ cup fat-free sour cream
> 2 tablespoons fat-free mayonnaise
> ½ teaspoon onion powder
> ¼ teaspoon garlic powder
> 1 can (16 ounces) peach halves (packed in juice), drained
> 2 tablespoons grated Parmesan cheese

1. Bring about an inch of water to a boil in a large skillet over high heat. Carefully add the turkey. Cover, reduce the heat to medium-low, and simmer for 15 to 20 minutes, or until the pieces are no longer pink in the center when cut with a sharp knife. Cook the broccoli according to the package directions.

2. In a small bowl, mix the sour cream, mayonnaise, onion powder, and garlic powder.

3. Preheat the broiler. Coat a shallow baking pan with cooking spray. Add the turkey, then arrange the broccoli and peaches around the tenderloins. Spoon the sour cream mixture on top and sprinkle with the cheese.

4. Broil 6" to 7" from the heat for 5 to 6 minutes, or until the sour cream mixture is puffy and lightly browned.

Makes 4 servings

Per serving: 253 calories, 3 g fat, 71 mg cholesterol, 5 g fiber, 277 mg sodium

Chicken Roasted with Winter Vegetables

This chicken is stuffed with vegetables instead of a high-calorie bread dressing. It would go especially well with a rice or barley pilaf.

1 broiler-fryer chicken (about 3 pounds)

1 clove garlic, finely chopped

4 sprigs fresh rosemary

4 small potatoes, quartered

3 medium carrots, halved and quartered

1 small onion, quartered

1 small fennel bulb, chopped

½ cup water

1. Preheat the oven to 400°F.

2. Rinse the chicken with cold water and pat dry with paper towels. Remove any excess fat from inside the chicken. Starting at the neck opening, use your fingers to gently loosen the skin from the meat to create a pocket on each side of the breast. Leave the skin attached to the breast bones.

3. Rub the garlic onto the meat underneath the skin. Then place the rosemary underneath the skin. Place the chicken, breast side up, on a rack in a shallow roasting pan. Loosely stuff with some of the potatoes, carrots, onion, and fennel. Place the remaining vegetables in the pan around the chicken. Skewer the neck skin to the back of the chicken and tie the legs to the tail. Insert a meat thermometer in the thickest part of a thigh. Pour the water in the bottom of the pan.

4. Roast for 30 minutes. Turn the vegetables over and roast for 30 minutes, or until the thermometer registers 180° to 185°.

5. Transfer the vegetables to a serving dish and keep warm. Loosely cover the chicken with foil and let stand for 10 minutes before carving. Remove and discard the skin before eating.

Makes 6 servings

Per serving: 188 calories, 4 g fat, 79 mg cholesterol, 2 g fiber, 129 mg sodium

Georgian Split Pea Soup

The Georgia referred to here is in Russia, where a low-cost soup like this would be standard peasant fare. But there's nothing commonplace about the robust flavor of this filling soup.

1	large tomato, chopped
3	cups water
1	large carrot, sliced diagonally
½	cup shredded cabbage
¼	cup dried yellow split peas, sorted and rinsed
¼	cup pearl barley
2	tablespoons finely chopped parsley
1	teaspoon reduced-sodium soy sauce
1	clove garlic, finely chopped

1. Place the tomato and 1 cup of the water in a blender. Process until smooth. Transfer to a large saucepan. Add the carrot, cabbage, split peas, barley, parsley, soy sauce, garlic, and the remaining 2 cups water.

2. Cover and bring to a boil over high heat. Reduce the heat to medium and simmer for 1¼ hours, or until the barley is tender.

Makes 4 servings

Per serving: 105 calories, 0.5 g fat, 0 mg cholesterol, 3 g fiber, 70 mg sodium

Note: Unlike most other legumes, split peas don't need to be soaked before being cooked. Simply rinse them well and pick them over to remove any small stones or other debris.

Curried Lentil Soup

Here's a tasty way to add fiber to your diet. If desired, serve with a dollop of fat-free plain yogurt in each bowlful.

½	cup chopped onion
½	cup chopped celery
½	cup chopped carrot
3	cups water
1	can (16 ounces) low-sodium tomatoes (with juice), cut up
¾	cup lentils, sorted and rinsed
2	teaspoons curry powder

1. Place the onion, celery, carrot, and 1 cup of the water in a blender. Process until smooth. Transfer to a large saucepan.

2. Add the tomatoes (with juice), lentils, curry powder, and the remaining 2 cups water. Cover and bring to a boil over high heat. Reduce the heat to medium and simmer for 1 hour.

Makes 4 servings

Per serving: 166 calories, 1 g fat, 0 mg cholesterol, 7 g fiber, 53 mg sodium

Note: Unlike most other legumes, lentils don't need to be soaked before being cooked. Simply rinse them well and pick them over to remove any small stones or other debris.

Sourdough Bread

You have to think ahead to make this bread because the starter needs 5 days to age properly—and you need enough friends and family to share it with! But it's well worth the effort.

Sourdough Starter

1	package active dry yeast
1	teaspoon sugar
1–1½	cups warm water (105°–115°F)
2	cups all-purpose flour

Bread Dough

1	cup warm water (105°–115°F)
2	teaspoons salt
4½–5	cups bread flour

1. *To make the sourdough starter:* In a large bowl, mix the yeast, sugar, water, and flour. Loosely cover and let stand in a warm place for 5 days, stirring at least once a day. When the starter is ready for use, it will be bubbly and may have a layer of yellow liquid on top. Stir well before using.

2. *To make the bread dough:* Add the water, salt, and 1 cup of the flour into the starter and stir. Gradually stir in enough of the remaining flour to make a very stiff dough. Turn the dough out onto a lightly floured surface and knead until the dough is smooth and elastic, adding flour as needed. (You may also turn the dough into the bowl of a heavy-duty mixer with a dough hook and knead for 8 to 10 minutes, or until the dough is smooth and elastic.)

3. Coat a clean large bowl with cooking spray. Place the dough in the bowl, cover with a damp towel, and let rise in a warm place for 2 hours, or until the dough is doubled in volume. At this point, you may use all of the dough to make one loaf of bread or remove some of the dough to repeat the starter process so you can make more loaves of bread in the future (see note).

4. Shape the dough into a round loaf about 2½" thick. Coat a nonstick baking sheet with cooking spray. Place the loaf on the sheet. Loosely cover with a damp cloth and let rise for 1 to 2 hours, or until the dough is doubled in volume.

5. Preheat the oven to 400°F. With a sharp knife, make three ¼"-deep slits on the top of the loaf. Bake for 20 to 25 minutes, or until golden and crusty. Cool on a rack.

Makes 24 slices

Per slice: 106 calories, 0 g fat, 0 mg cholesterol, 1 g fiber, 178 mg sodium

Note: To save some starter, remove 1 cup of the risen dough and place it in a plastic bowl with a tight-fitting lid. Pour 1½ cups warm water over the dough. Stir in 1 cup all-purpose flour. Cover and let stand at room temperature until the starter has doubled in volume. Then cover and refrigerate until you are ready to bake again.

If you don't plan to make bread again within a week, you can refrigerate the starter indefinitely by refreshing it once a week. To do this, remove and discard 1 cup of the starter. Into the remaining starter, stir 1½ cups warm water and 1 cup all-purpose flour. Cover and let stand at room temperature until the starter has doubled. Refrigerate for 1 week. Repeat until you are ready to make bread.

Variations

■ Sourdough Hard Rolls: Divide the risen dough into 12 equal-size pieces. Coat a nonstick baking sheet with cooking spray. Place the dough pieces on the baking sheet. Cover with a damp cloth and let rise in a warm place for 1 to 2 hours, or until doubled in volume. Bake at 400°F for 12 to 15 minutes or until golden.

■ Sourdough Breadsticks: Divide the risen dough in half. Divide each half into 32 equal-size pieces. Shape each piece into an 8"-long breadstick. Coat 2 nonstick baking sheets with cooking spray. Place the dough pieces on the baking sheets. Lightly brush the breadsticks with beaten egg white and sprinkle with sesame seeds. Cover with a damp cloth and let rise in a warm place for 30 minutes or until doubled in volume. Bake at 400°F for 15 minutes, or until golden.

Pesto

Fresh basil is generally available year-round in the produce section of the supermarket. Toss this delicious Italian paste with hot pasta, spread on toasted slices of Italian bread, or use as a baked-potato topping.

2¼   cups fresh basil leaves
¼   cup toasted walnuts
¼   cup scallions cut into 1" pieces
2   tablespoons lemon juice
2   cloves garlic
¼   teaspoon freshly ground black pepper
¾   cup fat-free, reduced-sodium chicken broth
3   tablespoons grated reduced-fat Parmesan cheese

1. Place the basil in a food processor or blender. Process until finely chopped. Add the walnuts, scallions, lemon juice, garlic, and pepper. Process until the walnuts are finely chopped.

2. With the motor running, gradually add the broth and cheese, blending until well-mixed.

Makes ⅔ cup

Per 2 tablespoons: 58 calories, 4 g fat, 0 mg cholesterol, 1 g fiber, 106 mg sodium

Note: Pesto can be frozen in airtight containers for up to 3 months.

Variation

■ Mixed Herb Pesto: Replace the basil with ¾ cup Italian parsley, ¾ cup fresh dill, and ¾ cup fresh basil leaves.

You're from a culture where food is equated with love.

What you need: low-fat ethnic favorites

The next time your well-meaning but food-pushing Aunt Ida or Bubie urges you to have "just a taste" of one of her traditional ethnic dishes, you can resist, knowing that you can make these scrumptious-but-slimmed-down versions of Italian, Greek, and Jewish meals at home.

COMMONSENSE STRATEGY: You know the line: "I made this just for you . . . eat, eat!" While these ethnic specialties are healthier and lower in calories than many, remember: Portion control, portion control, portion control.

Creamy Caprese Pasta

This Italian-style pasta dish tastes like pesto, but it's creamier. Calcium-rich yogurt is the secret and one of the reasons why this recipe is bone healthy.

1	pound whole wheat pasta, such as twists
1	cup fat-free plain yogurt
4	teaspoons extra-virgin olive oil
½	teaspoon salt
1	clove garlic
1	cup packed fresh basil leaves
2	tomatoes, chopped
1	teaspoon balsamic or red wine vinegar
6	ounces reduced-fat mozzarella cheese, cubed

1. Prepare the pasta according to package directions. Drain and return to the pot.
2. Place the yogurt, oil, salt, and garlic in a blender. Blend until smooth. Add the basil and blend well. Pour over the pasta and mix well.
3. Place the tomatoes in a small bowl. Toss with the vinegar and add the cheese. Serve over the pasta.

Makes 5 servings

Per serving: 475 calories, 11 g fat, 20 mg cholesterol, 11 g fiber, 418 mg sodium

Focaccia Bread with Marinated Vegetables

Bright vegetables and mellow cheese are sandwiched in focaccia bread,
which absorbs the flavors of their marinade.

1   jar (3½ ounces) chopped roasted red bell peppers, drained
3   cups thickly sliced mushrooms
1   tablespoon pitted and chopped black olives
1   teaspoon drained capers
2   tablespoons balsamic vinegar
1   tablespoon olive oil
1   clove garlic, finely chopped
    Salt
    Freshly ground black pepper
1   loaf focaccia bread
2   ounces reduced-fat mozzarella cheese, thinly sliced

1. In a large bowl, mix the red peppers, mushrooms, olives, and capers.

2. In a cup, whisk together the vinegar, oil, and garlic. Pour over the vegetables and toss to coat. Season with the salt and black pepper.

3. Cut the focaccia bread in half horizontally. Cover the bottom half with the vegetable mixture and sprinkle with the cheese. Add the top of the focaccia bread and press firmly. Cut into quarters.

Makes 4 servings

Per serving: 476 calories, 16.5 g fat, 5 mg cholesterol, 4 g fiber, 363 mg sodium

Italian Nachos

Here's the best of two cultures!

    3   whole wheat pitas
    1   cup shredded fat-free or reduced-fat mozzarella cheese
    1   tablespoon grated Parmesan cheese
    1   teaspoon dried basil
    1   teaspoon dried oregano
    ½   teaspoon dried thyme
    ¼   teaspoon paprika
    ¼   teaspoon freshly ground black pepper

1. Preheat the oven to 350°F. Line 2 large baking sheets with foil, then coat with cooking spray.

2. Cut each pita into 1½" triangles. Then split each triangle to form 2 layers. Place on the baking sheets in a single layer.

3. In a small bowl, mix the mozzarella cheese, Parmesan cheese, basil, oregano, thyme, paprika, and pepper. Sprinkle over the pita pieces.

4. Bake for 10 to 15 minutes, or until the pitas are golden and the cheese is melted.

Makes 4 servings

Per serving: 89 calories, 1 g fat, 6 mg cholesterol, 1 g fiber, 430 mg sodium

Zuccotto

Substitute orange juice for the Marsala if you prefer to omit the alcohol.

1	container (32 ounces) low-fat vanilla yogurt
½	cup confectioners' sugar
1	square (1 ounce) semisweet chocolate, finely chopped
¼	cup blanched slivered almonds
1	fat-free pound cake (13.6 ounces)
2	tablespoons orange juice
2	tablespoons sweet Marsala wine
1	envelope unflavored gelatin
¼	cup cold water

1. Line a strainer with a double layer of paper towels and place over a medium bowl. Spoon in the yogurt and let drain for 4 hours. Discard the liquid that drains and spoon the yogurt into the bowl. Stir in the confectioners' sugar and chocolate.

2. Preheat the oven to 350°F. Place the almonds in a baking pan and toast for about 8 minutes, or until lightly browned. Chop and stir into the yogurt.

3. Coat a deep 8-cup bowl with cooking spray. Line the bowl with plastic wrap. Cut the pound cake into twenty ¼"-thick slices. Place one whole slice of cake in the center of the bottom of the bowl. Cut the remaining slices in half diagonally. Arrange enough cake triangles around the inside of the bowl to cover the bowl, overlapping to fit.

4. In a cup, combine the orange juice and Marsala. Brush over the cake slices.

5. In a small saucepan, sprinkle the gelatin over the water and let stand for 1 minute. Cook over low heat, stirring, for 2 to 3 minutes, or until the gelatin dissolves. Gradually whisk into the yogurt, whisking constantly until it is completely incorporated.

6. Gently spoon the yogurt mixture into the bowl to cover the cake. Cover the yogurt mixture completely with the remaining cake slices. Brush the remaining orange juice mixture onto the cake slices. Cover with plastic wrap and chill for at least 3 hours.

7. To serve, uncover and invert the zuccotto onto a platter. Remove the bowl and plastic wrap.

Makes 12 servings

Per serving: 183 calories, 3.5 g fat, 2 mg cholesterol, 1 g fiber, 137 mg sodium

Mediterranean Shrimp with Feta

This is a favorite Greek way of preparing shrimp. Serve with French or Italian bread or warm pita pockets.

1	pound potatoes, peeled and thinly sliced
½	pound green beans, halved
1	medium zucchini, halved lengthwise and thinly sliced
2	teaspoons olive oil
1	onion, thinly sliced
1	red bell pepper, coarsely chopped
2	cloves garlic, finely chopped
1	can (28 ounces) crushed tomatoes (with juice)
1	pound shrimp, peeled and deveined
¼	cup dry white wine
½	teaspoon dried oregano
½	teaspoon salt
¼	teaspoon freshly ground black pepper
2	ounces feta cheese, crumbled
3	tablespoons chopped parsley

1. Preheat the oven to 375°F.

2. Place the potatoes in a large saucepan and add water to cover. Bring to a boil and cook for 7 minutes. Add the beans and zucchini. Cook for 3 minutes. Drain and transfer to a large bowl.

3. Warm the oil in a nonstick skillet over medium heat. Add the onion, bell pepper, and garlic. Cook for 3 minutes, or until softened. Add to the other vegetables.

4. Gently stir in the tomatoes (and juice), shrimp, wine, oregano, salt, and black pepper. Transfer to an 11" × 7" baking dish, cover with foil, and bake for 25 minutes.

5. Uncover and sprinkle the cheese on top. Bake, uncovered, for 3 minutes. Remove from the oven and sprinkle with the parsley.

Makes 4 servings

Per serving: 309 calories, 8 g fat, 152 mg cholesterol, 5 g fiber, 904 mg sodium

Greek Skillet Dinner in a Pita

Resembling an exotic street snack more than a traditional skillet dinner, this delicious lamb-and-eggplant mixture is served in pitas.

4	teaspoons olive oil
1	pound eggplant, cut into ¾" cubes
¼	cup fat-free, reduced-sodium chicken broth
¾	pound lean boneless leg of lamb, cut into ½" cubes
1	onion, chopped
2	ribs celery, diced
3	cloves garlic, finely chopped
2	teaspoons ground cumin
½	teaspoon dried oregano
¼	teaspoon dried mint
¼	teaspoon salt
¼	teaspoon freshly ground black pepper
1	can (14½ ounces) diced tomatoes (with juice)
1	can (10 ounces) chickpeas, rinsed and drained
4	pitas, halved
½	cup fat-free plain yogurt
4	cups shredded romaine lettuce
1	cup sliced peeled cucumbers
2	plum tomatoes, thinly sliced

1. Warm 2 teaspoons of the oil in a large skillet over medium-high heat. Add the eggplant and cook for 3 minutes, or until browned. Stir in the broth and bring to a boil. Reduce the heat to medium and cook for 5 minutes, or until the eggplant is tender and the liquid is absorbed. Transfer to a large plate.

2. Place the lamb in a food processor and process until coarsely ground.

3. Add the remaining 2 teaspoons oil to the skillet. Add the onion, celery, and garlic. Cook over medium-high heat for 3 minutes, or until the onion is tender. Crumble in the ground lamb and cook, stirring, for 3 minutes, or until the meat is no longer pink. Stir in the cumin, oregano, mint, salt, and pepper. Cook, stirring constantly, for 30 seconds.

4. Add the tomatoes (and juice) and bring to a boil. Stir in the chickpeas and reserved eggplant. Reduce the heat to low and simmer, stirring occasionally, for 5 minutes.

5. Serve spooned into the pitas. Top with the yogurt, lettuce, cucumbers, and plum tomatoes.

Makes 4 servings

Per serving: 475 calories, 11 g fat, 55 mg cholesterol, 8 g fiber, 851 mg sodium

Matzo Ball Soup

We updated these matzo balls by using egg whites and a reduced amount of oil. The soup is simple and flavorful, and the matzo balls are so tender.

4 egg whites

1 tablespoon canola oil

⅓ cup matzo meal

3 carrots, sliced

6 cups fat-free, reduced-sodium chicken broth

2 tablespoons chopped parsley

Pinch of freshly ground black pepper

1. Place the egg whites in a large bowl. Beat with an electric mixer until foamy. Beat in the oil and matzo meal. Cover and refrigerate for 20 minutes. Shape the mixture into 6 balls.

2. Bring a large pot of water to a boil over high heat. Carefully drop the matzo balls into the water. Add the carrots. Reduce the heat to medium-low, cover, and simmer for 30 minutes.

3. Drain the mixture, returning the carrots and matzo balls to the pot. Add the broth and cook over medium heat until heated through. Sprinkle with the parsley and season with the pepper.

Makes 6 servings

Per serving: 98 calories, 3 g fat, 0 mg cholesterol, 1 g fiber, 114 mg sodium

Beef and Mushroom Barley

Beef and barley are traditional Hanukkah foods. One way to keep beef dishes low in fat is by using lean cuts such as top round or eye of round.

2	cups water
2	cups fat-free, reduced-sodium beef broth
1	cup pearl barley
1	teaspoon dried thyme
2	cloves garlic, finely chopped
1	teaspoon olive oil
6	ounces boneless lean beef top round or eye of round, cut into ½" cubes
2	cups quartered mushrooms
1	cup chopped scallions
1	cup thinly sliced carrot
1	cup chopped celery
1½	cups vegetable juice cocktail
½	cup chopped tomatoes

1. In a medium saucepan, combine the water, broth, barley, thyme, and garlic. Bring to a boil, then reduce the heat. Simmer for 20 minutes.

2. Coat a large skillet with cooking spray. Add the oil and warm over medium-high heat. Add the beef. Stir for 5 minutes, or until the beef is lightly browned.

3. Add the mushrooms, scallions, carrot, and celery to the skillet. Stir for 3 minutes, or until the vegetables are crisp-tender.

4. Drain the barley and discard the liquid. Add the barley to the skillet. Stir in the vegetable juice and tomatoes. Cover and simmer for 15 to 20 minutes, or until the barley is just tender and the beef is cooked through.

Makes 4 servings

Per serving: 347 calories, 5 g fat, 38 mg cholesterol, 12 g fiber, 422 mg sodium

Baked Vegetable Latkes

Potato pancakes are a hallmark of Hanukkah, the Feast of Lights. Usually, they're fried in oil, but here we've baked them to cut back on fat. And we've given them a nutrient boost by adding carrots, zucchini, and parsnips.

1	large potato, peeled
2	medium carrots, peeled
1	small zucchini
1	small parsnip, peeled
1	small onion
½	cup fat-free liquid egg substitute
1½	tablespoons all-purpose flour
½	teaspoon baking powder
¼	teaspoon freshly ground black pepper

1. Preheat the oven to 425°F. Coat 2 large baking sheets with cooking spray.

2. Use a food processor to finely shred the potato, carrots, zucchini, parsnip, and onion. Squeeze any excess liquid from the vegetables and transfer to a large bowl. Stir in the egg substitute, flour, baking powder, and pepper. Mix well.

3. Using a tablespoon, spoon the batter onto the prepared baking sheets. Flatten each latke slightly with the back of the spoon. Bake for 10 to 15 minutes, or until golden.

Makes 4 servings

Per serving: 97 calories, 0 g fat, 0 mg cholesterol, 4 g fiber, 101 mg sodium

You're a chocolate addict.

What you need: low-fat chocolate treats

If you've got a "chocolate tooth," you probably already know that sometimes you just have to give in to temptation. But you don't have to jeopardize your weight-control program to do it. Make these chocolaty desserts only if you can eat them *in moderation*—that is, have one serving, not seven—and savor your favorite treat without sabotaging your program.

COMMONSENSE STRATEGY: Chewing gum as you bake is a great way to keep yourself from tasting the batter.

Chocolate Oatmeal Cookies

These are a new twist on an old favorite and have everything the originals do except the fat.

- ½ cup whole wheat flour
- ½ cup all-purpose flour
- 3 tablespoons unsweetened cocoa powder
- 1 teaspoon baking powder
- ½ teaspoon baking soda
- ½ teaspoon salt
- ½ teaspoon ground cinnamon
- ¼ cup unsweetened applesauce
- ¼ cup canola oil
- ½ cup packed brown sugar
- ¾ cup confectioners' sugar
- 1 large egg
- 1 teaspoon vanilla extract
- 1¼ cups rolled oats
- ½ cup raisins or chopped dates

1. Preheat the oven to 350°F. Coat baking sheets with cooking spray.

2. In a small bowl, mix the whole wheat flour, all-purpose flour, cocoa powder, baking powder, baking soda, salt, and cinnamon.

3. In a large bowl, mix the applesauce, oil, brown sugar, confectioners' sugar, egg, and vanilla. Add the flour mixture and mix well. Stir in the oats and raisins or dates. Drop by rounded teaspoonfuls onto the prepared baking sheets, leaving 2" between cookies.

4. Bake for 10 to 12 minutes, or until very lightly browned. Do not overbake. Remove the cookies to a rack to cool.

Makes 40

Per cookie: 57 calories, 2 g fat, 0 mg cholesterol, 1 g fiber, 47 mg sodium

Chocolate Crêpes with Berries

Along the streets of Paris, you'll find walk-up crêpe stands where Parisians buy crêpes-to-go. Serve this elegant fruit-filled version at a brunch, shower, or summertime tea.

½   **cup all-purpose flour**

2   **tablespoons unsweetened cocoa powder**

½   **cup fat-free milk**

2   **eggs**

2   **tablespoons honey**

2   **cups frozen fat-free vanilla yogurt**

2   **cups berries**

1. In a medium bowl, whisk together the flour and cocoa powder. Whisk in the milk, eggs, and honey. The batter should be the consistency of heavy cream. If necessary, thin with a little more milk. Let stand for 30 minutes.

2. Coat a medium nonstick skillet with cooking spray. Warm over medium heat. Add about 3 tablespoons of the batter and swirl to coat the bottom of the pan. Cook the crêpe for 1 minute, or until it easily comes loose from the pan. Turn and cook the other side for 30 seconds. Transfer to a plate.

3. Repeat to use all the batter.

4. To serve, place a small scoop of the frozen yogurt on each crêpe and roll to enclose the filling. Sprinkle with the berries.

Makes 4 servings

Per serving: 266 calories, 3.5 g fat, 109 mg cholesterol, 2 g fiber, 124 mg sodium

Chocolate-Walnut Biscotti

Dark and rich-tasting, these biscotti keep well in an airtight container or in the freezer. They are especially good dunked in espresso.

- 1 cup all-purpose flour
- ½ cup sugar
- ¼ cup unsweetened cocoa powder
- ½ teaspoon baking powder
- ¼ teaspoon baking soda
- ¼ teaspoon salt
- 1 egg
- 1 egg white
- 1½ teaspoons vanilla extract
- 2 ounces bittersweet chocolate, chopped
- ¼ cup chopped toasted walnuts (see note)

1. Preheat the oven to 350°F. Coat an 11" × 7" baking dish with cooking spray.
2. In a large bowl, whisk together the flour, sugar, cocoa powder, baking powder, baking soda, and salt.
3. In a medium bowl, whisk together the egg, egg white, and vanilla. Pour over the flour mixture and stir well. Stir in the chocolate and walnuts.
4. Press the dough into the baking dish. Bake for 25 minutes, or until firm. Transfer to a rack and cut into 30 fingers. Cool before serving.

Makes 30

Per biscotti: 75 calories, 3 g fat, 12 mg cholesterol, 1 g fiber, 44 mg sodium

Note: To toast nuts, spread them on a baking sheet and bake at 400°F for 10 minutes, or until lightly browned and fragrant. Do not let them burn.

Chocolate Indulgences

These little cupcakes make portion control easier.

4	squares (1 ounce each) semisweet chocolate
⅓	cup unsweetened cocoa powder
¾	cup sugar
½	cup evaporated fat-free milk
2	egg yolks
½	teaspoon vanilla extract
3	egg whites
¼	cup all-purpose flour
½	teaspoon baking powder
12	strawberries

1. Preheat the oven to 350°F. Line a 12-cup muffin pan with foil liners.

2. Place the chocolate in a large microwaveable bowl. Microwave on high power for 2 minutes to melt. Stir until smooth.

3. In a small saucepan, whisk together the cocoa and ½ cup of the sugar. Whisk in the milk. Cook for 2 minutes over medium heat, whisking constantly, until smooth. Stir the cocoa mixture into the melted chocolate. Stir in the egg yolks and vanilla extract.

4. Place the egg whites in a clean large bowl. Using an electric mixer, beat on medium speed until foamy. Gradually beat in the remaining ¼ cup sugar. Increase the speed to high and beat just until stiff. Use a rubber spatula to fold the egg whites into the chocolate mixture one-third at a time. Fold in the flour and baking powder.

5. Divide the batter evenly among the muffin cups. Bake for 20 to 22 minutes, or until a wooden pick inserted into the center comes out clean. Cool.

6. Top each cake with a strawberry.

Makes 12 servings

Per serving: 133 calories, 4 g fat, 36 mg cholesterol, 1 g fiber, 43 mg sodium

Banana-Chocolate Shake

When you have extra bananas on hand, slice and freeze them so that you can make this shake at a moment's notice.

1	small ripe banana
½	cup frozen fat-free chocolate or chocolate ripple yogurt
¼	teaspoon vanilla extract
⅔–¾	cup fat-free milk

1. Slice the banana and place the pieces in a small plastic bag. Close the bag and freeze for at least 1 hour, or until the pieces are solid.

2. Transfer the pieces to a food processor. Add the frozen yogurt, vanilla, and ⅔ cup of the milk. Process with on/off turns until smooth. (If the mixture is too thick to process easily, gradually add enough of the remaining milk to slightly thin it.)

Makes 1 serving

Per serving: 246 calories, 1 g fat, 3 mg cholesterol, 2 g fiber, 155 mg sodium

Easy Chocolate Pudding

Nobody will ever guess there's tofu behind this rich and creamy pudding.

1	package (12.3 ounces) light silken tofu
1	package (1.4 ounces) instant sugar-free chocolate pudding mix
⅔	cup dry milk
1	cup prepared coffee, cold
1	teaspoon coconut extract (optional)
1	cup frozen fat-free whipped topping, thawed
1	tablespoon finely chopped pecans (optional)

1. Place the tofu in a blender and process until smooth. Add the pudding mix, dry milk, coffee, and coconut extract (if using). Blend until smooth, scraping down the sides of the container as necessary. Transfer to a bowl. Fold in ¾ cup of the whipped topping.

2. Divide among 6 dishes. Chill for 30 minutes. Garnish with pecans (if using) and the remaining whipped topping.

Makes six ½-cup servings

Per ½ cup: 100 calories, 2 g fat, 1 mg cholesterol, 0 g fiber, 157 mg sodium

Chocolate Frozen Yogurt Pops

This is an inexpensive version of the frozen yogurt pops you find in the supermarket. For fruit pops, use strawberry or raspberry syrup instead of the chocolate.

1 **cup fat-free plain yogurt**
3 **tablespoons light corn syrup**
2 **tablespoons chocolate syrup**
½ **teaspoon vanilla extract**
⅔ **cup 2% milk**

1. In a small bowl, mix the yogurt and corn syrup. Stir in the chocolate syrup and vanilla. Add the milk and mix well.

2. Pour the mixture into eight 6-ounce ice-pop molds or paper cups, filling each about three-quarters full. Cover the molds with their lids or the paper cups with foil. Insert the sticks (use wooden ice-pop sticks if using paper cups). Freeze until solid. To serve, remove the pops from the mold according to the directions that came with it or peel the paper from the cups.

Makes 8

Per pop: 60 calories, 0.5 g fat, 2 mg cholesterol, 0 g fiber, 40 mg sodium

Chocolate Soufflés

Chocoholics will love this one! These individual soufflés are so rich in chocolate flavor that it's hard to believe they have only 136 calories.

¼   **cup unsweetened cocoa powder**

2   **tablespoons cornstarch**

1   **teaspoon ground cinnamon**

¾   **cup milk**

½   **cup reduced-calorie maple-flavored syrup**

2   **egg yolks**

3   **egg whites**

½   **teaspoon cream of tartar**

1. Preheat the oven to 400°F. Coat six 6-ounce soufflé dishes or custard cups with cooking spray.

2. In a medium saucepan, mix the cocoa powder, cornstarch, and cinnamon. Stir in the milk and maple syrup. Stir over medium heat for 4 to 8 minutes or until heated through.

3. Place the egg yolks in a small bowl and beat lightly. Slowly stir about one-quarter of the hot cocoa mixture into the egg yolks. Then stir the yolk mixture into the saucepan. Set aside.

4. Place the egg whites in a large bowl. Add the cream of tartar. Using an electric mixer, beat on high speed until the egg whites form soft peaks. Gently fold one-quarter of the egg whites into the cocoa mixture. Then gently fold in the remaining egg whites. Spoon the mixture evenly into the prepared cups.

5. Place the cups on a baking sheet. Bake for 15 to 20 minutes, or until the soufflés are puffed and a knife inserted near the center comes out clean. Serve immediately.

Makes 6 servings

Per serving: 136 calories, 3 g fat, 73 mg cholesterol, 0 g fiber, 50 mg sodium

Banana Ice Cream
with Silky Chocolate Sauce

This tastes like premium ice cream with only a fraction of the fat.

Ice Cream

2   large ripe frozen bananas, sliced

2   tablespoons sugar

1½   cups 1% milk

½   teaspoon ground cinnamon

½   teaspoon vanilla extract

Chocolate Sauce

⅔   cup water

¼   cup sugar

3   tablespoons unsweetened cocoa powder

2   teaspoons cornstarch

2   teaspoons unsalted butter

½   teaspoon vanilla extract

1. *To make the ice cream:* Combine the bananas, sugar, and ½ cup of the milk in a blender. Process until smooth. Add the cinnamon, vanilla, and the remaining 1 cup milk. Process until smooth. Transfer into an 8" × 8" metal or plastic container. Cover and freeze for at least 4 hours.

2. Remove from the freezer and break up the mixture with a knife. Working with half of the mixture at a time, process briefly in a food processor or blender. The mixture will transform from icy to smooth. Use a rubber spatula to poke the mixture down. Return it to the container, cover, and freeze for at least 30 minutes before serving.

3. *To make the chocolate sauce:* In a medium saucepan, combine the water, sugar, cocoa powder, and cornstarch. Whisk until smooth. Cook over medium heat, stirring frequently with a wooden spoon, for 5 minutes, or until smooth and thickened. Remove from the heat and stir in the butter and vanilla. Serve warm or at room temperature over the ice cream. Store leftovers in the refrigerator.

Makes 6 servings

Per serving: 129 calories, 2.5 g fat, 6 mg cholesterol, 1 g fiber, 34 mg sodium

You stick to your diet Monday through Friday afternoon . . . and blow it over the weekend.

What you need: healthy weekend eats

All week, you resist the temptation of French toast, steak sandwiches, pizza, and fries. Now, you don't have to "just say no" during the weekend. These recipes leave in the decadence but remove one critical ingredient: guilt.

COMMONSENSE STRATEGY: Weekend meals can be more flexible than your Monday-through-Friday menus, but they still need to support your goals. So on the weekends, eat what you like . . . just rein it in a bit. Have two meals instead of three. Eat a piece of fruit or two in between. And designate one meal your "fun" meal but subtract calories from the other.

Orange-Sauced Crêpes

Any morning that starts with these crêpes is bound to be good!

Filling

- ¾ cup reduced-fat ricotta cheese
- ¼ cup raisins
- 1 tablespoon honey

Crêpes

- 2 egg whites, lightly beaten
- ¾ cup fat-free milk
- ½ cup whole wheat flour

Sauce

- 2 tablespoons water
- 2 teaspoons cornstarch
- 1 teaspoon grated orange peel

1   cup orange juice

1   teaspoon honey

1   can (10½ ounces) mandarin orange sections (packed in water), drained

1. *To make the filling:* In a small bowl, combine the ricotta cheese, raisins, and honey.

2. *To make the crêpes:* In a small bowl, combine the egg whites, milk, and flour. Whisk until smooth.

3. Coat a medium nonstick skillet with cooking spray. Warm over medium heat. Add about 2 tablespoons of the batter and swirl to coat the bottom of the pan. Cook the crêpe for 1 minute, or until it easily comes loose from the pan. Turn and cook the other side for 30 seconds. Transfer to a plate.

4. Repeat to use all the batter and make 8 crêpes.

5. Preheat the oven to 350°. Coat an 8" × 8" baking dish with cooking spray.

6. Spoon a rounded tablespoon of the filling mixture on the center of each crêpe. Form each into a packet by folding two opposite sides to the center, overlapping the edges slightly. Then fold in the remaining two sides.

7. Place the packets in the baking dish, overlapping slightly. Cover with foil and bake for 15 to 20 minutes, or until heated through.

8. *To make the sauce:* Mix the water and cornstarch in a small saucepan. Stir in the orange peel, orange juice, and honey. Stir over medium heat until the mixture thickens and begins to gently boil. Stir for 2 minutes. Gently stir in the oranges.

9. To serve, arrange 2 crêpes on each plate. Serve with the warm sauce.

Makes 4 servings

Per serving: 249 calories, 4.5 g fat, 15 mg cholesterol, 3 g fiber, 116 mg sodium

Note: Save time by making the crepes ahead. Let them cool, then stack the bunch and cover with plastic wrap. Refrigerate for up to 4 days. For longer storage, freeze the crêpes. They'll be easier to separate later if you place 2 pieces of waxed paper between each pair. Wrap airtight. When ready to use, thaw the crêpes in the refrigerator overnight or at room temperature until pliable.

Oven-Crisped French Toast with Apricot Sauce

*Egg whites and fat-free milk slim down this favorite considerably.
And baking rather than frying the bread slices in butter keeps the fat low.*

French Toast

4   egg whites
½   cup fat-free milk
½   teaspoon ground cinnamon
½   teaspoon vanilla extract
8   slices whole wheat bread

Sauce

2   tablespoons water
1½   teaspoons cornstarch
1   can (6 ounces) apricot nectar
1   tablespoon honey

1. *To make the French toast:* Preheat the oven to 450°F. Coat a baking sheet with cooking spray.

2. In a shallow bowl, beat together the egg whites, milk, cinnamon, and vanilla.

3. Dip the bread slices, one at a time, into the egg mixture, coating both sides. Place on the baking sheet.

4. Bake for 6 minutes. Turn the bread slices and bake for 5 minutes, or until golden brown.

5. *To make the sauce:* Mix the water and cornstarch in a small saucepan. Stir in the apricot nectar and honey. Stir over medium heat until the mixture thickens and begins to gently boil. Stir for 2 minutes. Serve over the French toast.

Makes 4 servings

Per serving: 205 calories, 2 g fat, 1 mg cholesterol, 3 g fiber, 289 mg sodium

Eggs Benedict with Almost Classic Hollandaise

The sauce tastes like the real thing! But unlike the original, which weighs in at a whopping 25 grams of fat, this version has only 4 grams per serving.

4	teaspoons unsalted butter
½	cup water
1	egg yolk
2½	teaspoons lemon juice
¾	teaspoon Dijon mustard
½	teaspoon salt
1¼	teaspoons all-purpose flour
½	teaspoon grated lemon peel
8	English muffin halves, toasted
4	slices Canadian bacon, cooked
4	poached eggs

1. Melt the butter in a small saucepan over medium heat.

2. Whisk the water, egg yolk, lemon juice, mustard, and salt in a small bowl. Gradually whisk in the flour.

3. Off heat, whisk the egg yolk mixture into the butter, stirring constantly. Still whisking, bring to a boil and simmer for 30 seconds. Remove from the heat and stir in the lemon peel.

4. Top each English muffin half with a slice of bacon and an egg. Drizzle with the sauce.

Makes 4 servings

Per serving: 320 calories, 12.5 g fat, 300 mg cholesterol, 0 g fiber, 1,203 mg sodium

Omelet in an English Muffin

No need to stop at a fast-food restaurant on the way to work. Here's a low-calorie, low-fat version of the popular egg 'n' muffin sandwich. For variety, replace the ham with cooked lean beef, chicken, or turkey breast.

½ cup fat-free liquid egg substitute

¼ cup water

½ teaspoon dried basil

⅓ cup finely chopped cooked lean ham

¼ cup sliced scallions

¼ cup shredded reduced-fat mozzarella cheese

⅓ cup fat-free ranch-style dressing

1 teaspoon mustard

5 whole wheat English muffins, split and toasted

1. Coat a large skillet with cooking spray. Warm over medium heat.

2. In a small bowl, beat together the egg substitute, water, and basil. Stir in the ham and scallions. Pour into the hot skillet and cook until the egg begins to set. Using a large spoon, lift and turn the egg mixture so it cooks evenly. Cook until the egg mixture is thoroughly cooked but still glossy and moist on top. Remove the skillet from the heat and sprinkle with the cheese.

3. In a small bowl, mix the dressing and mustard. Spread on the English muffin halves. Spoon the egg mixture onto half of the English muffins. Top with the remaining halves.

Makes 5 servings

Per serving: 190 calories, 2.5 g fat, 8 mg cholesterol, 1 g fiber, 632 mg sodium

Note: You can make these ahead, wrap individually, and store in the freezer. Thaw overnight in the refrigerator. Remove the freezer wrap and wrap each sandwich in foil. Bake at 350°F for 25 minutes, or until heated through. Or vent the freezer wrap and microwave each sandwich on medium power for 1 minute. Rotate the sandwich a half-turn. Microwave on medium power for ½ to 1 minute.

Seafood Paella

Here's a simplified version of a Spanish favorite. Besides being quicker to make, it's lower in fat and calories.

2 tablespoons olive oil	¼ teaspoon ground saffron or turmeric
1 tablespoon finely chopped garlic	1½ cups fat-free chicken broth
¾ pound shelled large shrimp	1 bottle (8 ounces) clam juice
2 tablespoons lemon juice	12 small clams, scrubbed
1 onion, finely chopped	1 cup frozen peas (thawed)
1 carrot, finely chopped	1 yellow or red bell pepper, finely chopped
1 cup brown rice	2 cups cherry tomatoes, halved
½ teaspoon salt	¼ cup finely chopped parsley
½ teaspoon dried oregano or thyme	6 pimiento-stuffed olives, thinly sliced
½ teaspoon ground paprika	

1. Heat 1 tablespoon of the oil in a large nonstick skillet over medium-high heat. Add the garlic and stir for 30 seconds. Add the shrimp and stir for 1 minute. Add the lemon juice and stir for 1 minute. Transfer the shrimp mixture to a plate.

2. Add the remaining 1 tablespoon oil to the skillet. Add the onion and cook for 3 minutes. Add the carrot and cook for 3 minutes. Add the rice and stir for 1 minute. Add the salt, oregano or thyme, paprika, saffron or turmeric, broth, and clam juice. Bring to a boil.

3. Cover tightly, reduce the heat to low, and simmer for 40 minutes. Arrange the clams around the edge of the skillet. Cover and cook for 15 minutes or until the rice is just tender and the broth is almost completely absorbed.

4. Slightly bury the shrimp in the rice. Sprinkle with the peas, bell pepper, and tomatoes. Cover and cook for 10 minutes, or until the vegetables and shrimp are heated through. Sprinkle with the parsley and olives.

Makes 4 servings

Per serving: 361 calories, 10 g fat, 47 mg cholesterol, 7 g fiber, 588 mg sodium

Texas Beef Soft Tacos

By using soft flour tortillas instead of fried corn shells, we cut fat on this Tex-Mex favorite.

¾ pound beef tenderloin, trimmed of all visible fat

1½ teaspoons ground cumin

¼ cup fat-free chicken broth

1 cup chopped red bell pepper

3 cloves garlic, finely chopped

2 canned chipotle chile peppers in adobo sauce, finely chopped

½ cup mild salsa

8 flour tortillas (12" diameter)

3 ounces shredded reduced-fat Monterey Jack cheese

¼ cup fat-free sour cream

¼ cup chopped cilantro

1. Cut the beef across the grain into very thin strips. Place in a large bowl, sprinkle with the cumin, and toss well.

2. Bring the broth to a boil in a large nonstick skillet over medium-high heat. Add the red pepper and garlic. Cook for 3 minutes. Transfer to a plate. Add the beef to the pan and cook for 5 minutes. Stir in the chile peppers, salsa, and the red pepper mixture. Cook for 2 minutes.

3. Wrap the tortillas in plastic wrap and microwave on high power for 1 minute. Divide the beef mixture among the tortillas, top with the cheese, sour cream, and cilantro. Roll up.

Makes 4 servings

Per serving: 372 calories, 10 g fat, 60 mg cholesterol, 12 g fiber, 942 mg sodium

Philadelphia Steak Sandwiches

Rocky Balboa, the boxer-hero of the movies, introduced millions of Americans to Philadelphia's beloved steak sandwich. This low-fat version features reduced-fat mozzarella and plenty of sautéed vegetables. If you're adventuresome, add zing with hot cherry peppers.

- 1 red bell pepper, diced
- 1 green bell pepper, diced
- 1 onion, diced
- 8 mushrooms, thinly sliced
- 2 tablespoons sliced garlic
- ¾ pound beef round tip steak, sliced paper thin (see note)
- ¼ cup ketchup
- 1 teaspoon dried oregano
- ¼ teaspoon freshly ground black pepper
- 1 cup shredded reduced-fat mozzarella cheese
- 4 steak rolls, split and warmed

1. Coat a large skillet with cooking spray and warm over medium-high heat for 2 minutes. Add the red pepper, green pepper, onion, and mushrooms. Stir for 5 minutes, or until browned.

2. Add the garlic and steak. Cook for 3 minutes, or until the steak is no longer pink. Stir in the ketchup, oregano, and black pepper. Sprinkle with the mozzarella. Cover and cook over low heat for 5 minutes, or until the mozzarella melts. Divide among the rolls.

Makes 4 servings

Per serving: 330 calories, 13 g fat, 74 mg cholesterol, 3 g fiber, 399 mg sodium

Note: Freezing the steak for about 20 minutes will firm it enough to make thin-slicing easier.

Oven Fries

Why give up french fries? Here's a low-fat version to satisfy those cravings.

1	tablespoon olive oil
1½	tablespoons chopped fresh thyme or rosemary
¼	teaspoon freshly ground black pepper
3	large baking potatoes

1. Preheat the oven to 475°F. Coat a jelly-roll pan with cooking spray.

2. In a large bowl, mix the oil, thyme or rosemary, and pepper.

3. Cut each potato lengthwise into ½"-thick wedges. Add to the oil mixture and toss to coat. Place the potatoes in a single layer on the prepared pan.

4. Bake, turning occasionally, for 15 to 20 minutes, or until the potatoes are lightly browned and tender.

Makes 4 servings

Per serving: 196 calories, 4 g fat, 0 mg cholesterol, 4 g fiber, 12 mg sodium

Variations

■ Crab-Boil Oven Fries: Replace the thyme and black pepper with 1 tablespoon crab-boil seasoning.

■ Southwest Oven Fries: Replace the thyme and black pepper with 1 teaspoon each ground cumin, chili powder, paprika, and dried oregano. Add ¼ teaspoon ground red pepper.

■ Spicy Oven Fries: Replace the thyme and black pepper with 1 tablespoon stone-ground mustard, 1 clove finely chopped garlic, 1 teaspoon dried tarragon, ¼ teaspoon paprika, and ⅛ teaspoon ground red pepper.

Greengrocer's Pizza

Bet you've never had this before. It's a fresh, crispy salad served up in a pizza shell. Popular in trattorias throughout Italy, its success relies on very fresh ingredients.

Crust

1   teaspoon cornmeal

1   pound refrigerated pizza dough

¼   cup shredded provolone cheese

Vegetable Topping

2   tablespoons olive oil

2   teaspoons chopped fresh oregano

1   teaspoon balsamic vinegar

1   teaspoon lemon juice

2   plum tomatoes, cubed

2   tablespoons chopped red onion

2   tablespoons chopped fresh basil

     Salt

     Freshly ground black pepper

6   cups mixed lettuce

1. *To make the crust:* Preheat the oven to 500°F. Sprinkle the cornmeal on a large baking sheet.

2. Divide the dough into 4 pieces and form each into a 6" round. Place on the prepared baking sheet. Prick the dough deeply all over with a fork.

3. Bake for 10 minutes, or until the crusts turn golden brown. Sprinkle with the cheese. Bake for 2 minutes. Remove from the oven.

4. *To make the vegetable topping:* In a large bowl, whisk together the oil, oregano, vinegar, and lemon juice. Stir in the tomatoes, onion, basil, salt, and pepper. Add the lettuce and toss to coat. Divide the mixture evenly over the crusts.

Makes 4 servings

Per serving: 354 calories, 11.5 g fat, 5 mg cholesterol, 5 g fiber, 344 mg sodium

Part 6

THE NO-BRAINER MENU PLANNER (AND OTHER TASTY TOOLS)

The No-Brainer Menu Planner

Ever wish you could go to the fridge, local fast-food or take-out place, or a restaurant and automatically make or order a healthy, low-calorie meal—without counting calories? Well, now you can. Because I believe in the power of tools, I wanted to devise a way to make meals into tools. Hence, the No-Brainer Menu Planner—a quick, easy way to just eat, without ever opening a calorie counter. It's based on two tools found in the Food Tools chapter—tool 11: Assemble an arsenal of 300-calorie meals and tool 12: Follow up with 700-calorie meals.

Following, you'll find 60 breakfasts, lunches, and dinners that contain approximately 300, 500, and 700 calories and that you can make at home or order out. Because the calories have already been calculated for you, all you have to do is determine the approximate number of calories you want to "spend" on a meal, decide whether you'll eat at home or dine out, and pick a meal.

I'm sure some of you will find not tallying up calories unusual, especially since some of my tools involve counting calories and the journal that accompanies this book includes a calorie-counting diary. But as I've said time and again, no tool works for everyone, and not everyone wants to count calories.

So I dedicate these menus to the folks who loathe that task—and to any of you who count calories but occasionally want a no-hassle way to stay within your daily allotment.

Twenty 300-Calorie Meals

BREAKFAST

At Home

- Cereal (any kind; check the label and measure out 150 calories' worth)
- ½ cup fat-free milk
- ½ banana or ¼ cup raisins

    OR

- ½ cinnamon-raisin bagel (2 ounces of a 4-ounce bagel)
- 1 ounce cream cheese
- ½ cup orange juice

    OR

- 1 fruit smoothie: In a blender, whip until smooth 1 cup low-fat fortified soy or cow's milk, 1½ cups frozen raspberries or strawberries (no sugar added), half of a banana, ¼ cup light tofu, and 1 teaspoon sugar.

At a Restaurant

- 2 poached eggs on a dry English muffin

    OR

- 1 large bowl of oatmeal with 1 tablespoon sugar or maple syrup
- ½ cup fat-free milk
- ¼ cup raisins

    OR

- 1 soft-boiled egg
- 2 slices bacon
- 1 slice toast with butter

At a Fast-Food or Take-Out Place

McDonald's

- 1 fat-free apple-bran muffin
- 1 cup fat-free milk

    OR

- 1 cup low-fat fruit yogurt
- 1 cup fruit salad

LUNCH

At Home

- 1 No-Brainer sandwich: 2 slices bread, 3 ounces lean deli meat (turkey or ham), lettuce, tomato, and mustard
- 1 piece fruit

  OR

- 1 cup leftover anything
- Salad dressed with balsamic vinegar and 1 tablespoon olive oil

At a Restaurant

- Salad with grilled chicken or tuna and low-fat dressing on the side
- BLT, no mayo

At a Fast-Food or Take-Out Place

Wendy's

- Grilled chicken sandwich

Deli

- Sandwich on regular-size bread with half the usual filling, mustard, and no cheese or mayo

  OR

- Dole Completes Light Caesar Salad Kit

DINNER

At Home

- 1 veggie burger on hamburger roll with lettuce, tomato, onion, and ketchup
- 2 cups broccoli, steamed

  OR

- 3 ounces salmon, halibut, or orange roughy, steamed or poached
- ½ cup cooked white or brown rice or whole wheat couscous
- 8 large asparagus spears, steamed
- 1 cup strawberries or 1 small apple

At a Restaurant

- Shrimp cocktail
- Salad with 2 tablespoons vinaigrette dressing on the side
- ½ plate pasta with marinara sauce

    OR

- 1 plate veggies, steamed, over ⅔ cup rice

At a Fast-Food or Take-Out Place

Chinese Restaurant

- 1 small entrée, steamed, with mini carton of rice

Boston Market

- ½ chicken breast, roasted with skin (remove skin before eating)
- Steamed vegetables

Twenty 500-Calorie Meals

<u>BREAKFAST</u>

At Home

- 2 frozen waffles
- 2 tablespoons maple syrup
- 1 cup fruit salad

    OR

- 2 eggs scrambled in 1 tablespoon butter
- ½ bagel (2 ounces of 4-ounce bagel) with 1 tablespoon cream cheese and 2 ounces smoked salmon

    OR

- ½ pink grapefruit
- Instant oatmeal, plain (2 packets) with 1 cup fat-free milk and ½ ounce raisins
- 2 slices whole wheat toast with 2 teaspoons margarine

At a Restaurant

- 2 eggs, fried
- English muffin or toast, dry
- 2 slices bacon

    OR

- ½ cantaloupe
- 2 small pancakes with 1 tablespoon syrup
- 3 slices bacon

At a Fast-Food or Take-Out Place

Hardee's

- 3 pancakes with 2 teaspoons margarine and 2 tablespoons syrup

McDonald's

- 2 pancakes with 1 tablespoon syrup
- 1 scrambled egg

LUNCH

At Home

- Large salad made with lettuce, tomato, carrots, cucumber, etc., with balsamic vinegar and 1 tablespoon olive oil
- 7 Morningstar Farms Chik Nuggets with ¼ cup ketchup
- ½ cup cooked white or brown rice

    OR

- PBJ sandwich (2 tablespoons peanut butter, 1 tablespoon jelly)
- 1 glass fat-free milk

    OR

- Tuna sandwich (3 ounces tuna with 1 tablespoon real mayonnaise)

At a Restaurant

- Salad with grilled chicken and 2 tablespoons vinaigrette dressing on the side

At a Fast-Food or Take-Out Place

McDonald's

- Hamburger and small fries

Pizza Hut

- 2 slices Thin n' Crispy Pizza (from a medium pie)
- 1 slice apple or cherry dessert pizza

DINNER

At Home

- 6 ounces skinless chicken breast, broiled
- 1 medium baked white or sweet potato
- 1 cup cooked spinach dressed with lemon juice
- 1 broiled tomato sprinkled with Parmesan cheese

OR

- 6 ounces salmon, poached, with lemon juice
- 2 small boiled potatoes with 2 teaspoons butter and parsley
- Steamed vegetables

OR

- 1 cup brown rice mixed with 1 cup beans and 1 cup steamed vegetables

At a Restaurant

- 8 ounces lobster meat
- 2 ears corn on the cob

OR

- 6 ounces trout fillet, grilled
- ½ cup cooked barley or other grain
- 1 cup steamed veggies
- 1 teaspoon margarine

At a Fast-Food or Take-Out Place

Taco Bell

- Taco salad with salsa without shell
- ½ portion Mexican rice

OR

- Grilled-cheese sandwich

Twenty 700-Calorie meals

BREAKFAST

Note: Unless you're eating brunch, there's no reason to eat a 700-calorie breakfast.

At Home

- ½ cup fruit salad
- 2 scrambled eggs
- 3 pancakes (4 inch) with 2 teaspoons margarine
- 2 turkey breakfast sausage links

   OR

- 1 cup fruit salad
- 2 croissants with 1 tablespoon butter or margarine

At a Restaurant

- 2 pieces French toast with 2 tablespoons syrup
- 2 turkey breakfast sausage links

   OR

- 1 Bloody Mary
- Eggs Benedict: 2 poached eggs with 2 slices ham on a dry English muffin, hollandaise sauce on the side (3 tablespoons)

At a Fast-Food or Take-Out Place

- 1 croissant with egg and cheese
- 1 cup fruit salad
- 2 sausage patties

LUNCH

At Home

- 1 cup of clear soup such as vegetarian vegetable or chicken or beef noodle
- Tuna sandwich (3 ounces tuna with 1 tablespoon real mayonnaise)
- 1 sweet pickle
- Baby carrots and celery slices with 2 tablespoons dip

OR

- 1 cup cold soup such as gazpacho or potato leek
- 3 ounces sliced roast beef on rye with mustard
- 1 cup of spinach, or other vegetable, cooked
- 1 cup fresh fruit compote

At a Restaurant

- 2 small slices whole wheat crust pizza topped with broccoli

  OR

- 1 cup chicken noodle soup
- Turkey club, mayo on the side (2 tablespoons)

  OR

- 2 small pieces quiche
- 1 cup broccoli, steamed
- Salad with 1 tablespoon dressing (balsamic vinegar and olive oil)

At a Fast-Food or Take-Out Place

Deli

- Tuna sandwich on regular bread

McDonald's

- McChicken sandwich

DINNER

At Home

- 2 low-calorie frozen meals
- Salad with low-calorie dressing

  OR

- 6 ounces flank steak (sauté in nonstick pan with salt, pepper, and garlic, if desired)
- 1 cup vegetables, steamed
- 1 glass wine
- ½ cup wild rice or other grain (without butter or cheese)

At a Restaurant

- Shrimp cocktail (3 ounces shrimp)
- ½ serving vegetarian lasagna
- 1 cup salad with 4 medium black olives and 2 teaspoons Italian dressing
- 6 ounces red wine

   OR

- ¼ cup guacamole and 13 tortilla chips (put on a plate before eating)
- 1 serving shrimp or chicken fajitas
- 12 ounces beer

   OR

- ½ order pasta with pesto sauce
- Salad with low-calorie dressing on the side

   OR

- 6 ounces sirloin steak, broiled
- 1 large baked potato with 1 tablespoon sour cream
- 1 cup broccoli and carrots, steamed
- Blueberry pie (⅙ of 8-inch pie)

   OR

- ½ serving veal cordon bleu
- 2 cups salad with 2 teaspoons honey-mustard dressing
- ½ cup rice

At a Fast-Food or Take-Out Place

McDonald's

- Chicken McGrill
- 1 packet mayonnaise
- 1 low-fat frozen yogurt milkshake

Angelic (and Devilish) 100-Calorie Snacks

L ooking for a treat that will set you back only 100 calories? Look no further. Here are nearly 100 of them. You'll notice, however, that they're divided into two categories. Choose a snack from the "I'm Wearing a Halo Today" category when you feel particularly strong and committed to your program or simply want to get in your daily servings of fruits, vegetables, or whole grains. But at those times when you can't eat another carrot, skip to the "I'm Feeling Devilish Today" category. There, you'll likely find the snack your soul cries out for . . . but in mini-portions.

I'm Wearing a Halo Today

Snack	Calories
Apple, 1	80
Apricots, 10 dried	83
Artichoke, globe, 1 steamed	60
Banana, 1 (try freezing it)	105
Berries, ½ cup, with ½ cup low-fat cottage cheese	110
Biscotti, 1 Pepperidge Farm	90
Blueberries, ½ cup fresh, with 1 string cheese (¾ oz)	109
Cappuccino with fat-free milk, large	about 100
Carrots, 2 large, with 2 Tbsp hummus	118
Carrots, 15 baby, with ¼ cup light sour cream dip mix	124
Cashews, 9	80
Cereal, 1 single-serving box (1 oz)	about 100
Cheese, 1 oz	74–113
Cheese, Laughing Cow Lite Cheese, 2 wedges	100

Snack	Calories
Cherries, 1/2 cup canned	68
Corn on the cob, 1	59
Cranberries, 1 oz dried	103
Figs, 1/2 cup canned in light syrup	87
Fruit cocktail, 1/2 cup	91
Gooseberries, 1/2 cup fresh	33
Grapes, 1 1/2 cups frozen	93
Kiwifruit, 1 medium	50
Kumquat, 1	12
Lycee, 1 fresh	20
Mango, 1 (7 oz)	135
Oatmeal, 1 individual package	110–170
Orange, 1	62
Papaya, 1/2	60
Peach, 1	42
Pear, 1	48
Persimmon, Japanese, 1/2 large	58
Pineapple chunks, 1 cup fresh	76
Pistachio nuts, 20	85
Plums, 2	90
Popcorn, 3 cups air-popped	93
Potato, 1/2 baked	72
Prunes, 5	100
Raisins, 1/4 cup	108
Shake made with low-fat chocolate soy milk, low-fat vanilla yogurt, peanut butter, and ice	120
Sherbet, sorbet, or ice, 1/2 cup	61–127
Shrimp cocktail: 2 oz shrimp and 2 Tbsp cocktail sauce	86
Soup, turkey noodle, 1 cup	68
Soup, vegetable, 1 cup	75

Snack	Calories
Tomatoes and cucumbers dipped in low-fat plain yogurt mixed with salad dressing	102
Tomato juice, 1½ cups	62
Virgin Mary, 12 oz	64
Watermelon, 1½ cups	75
Whole wheat pita, small, stuffed with lettuce, cucumber, tomatoes, and salsa	121
Yogurt, 8 oz fat-free fruit or plain	135

I'm Feeling Devilish Today

Snack	Calories
Animal crackers, ½ box Nabisco	116
Apple fritter, 1 oz	87
Beer, light, 12 oz	99
Beer, nonalcoholic, 12 oz	32
Berries, ½ cup, with 1 fat-free cookie	100
Blackberries, 1 cup	74
Cake, 1 knuckle's-width slice	100
Candy, 1 Ferrero Rocher	75
Cheese curls, 8	80
Chestnuts, 4	80
Chips, 11 plain baked tortilla	93
Chocolate chip cookies, 2 Famous Amos	75
Cocoa, low-cal prepared with water, 1 cup	64
Cookies, Oreos, 2	106
Crackers, Aak-Mak Armenian cracker bread	116
Crackers, Natural Rye Krisp, 3	90
Crackers, Reduced-Fat Triscuits, 6	102
Daiquiri, nonalcoholic made with fresh fruit	80–100
Drake's Ring Ding, ½	75
Egg cream, chocolate: mix 1 Tbsp chocolate syrup, 6 oz 1% milk, and 6 oz seltzer	125

Snack	Calories
Fruit salad, ½ cup with 2 Tbsp fat-free whipped topping	57–127
Gelatin, 1 Jell-O strawberry	75
Gelatin with fruit added, ½ cup	73
Graham crackers, chocolate, 6 (1½ sheets)	105
Graham crackers, whole wheat honey, 8 (2 sheets)	110
Hazelnuts, 6	90
Ice cream, ¼ cup Breyers Natural Vanilla and Chocolate	75
Ice cream, low-fat, ½ cup	80
Ice cream sandwich, ½	71
Ice milk, strawberry, ½ cup	122
Ice milk, vanilla or chocolate, ½ cup	93
Lady fingers, 2, spread with 1 Tbsp fat-free cream cheese and 2 tsp jam	85
Little Debbie Golden Cremes, ½	75
Macadamia nuts, 6	100
Oyster and soup crackers, 28 crackers, Krispy brand	98
Peanuts, ½-oz packet (17 nuts)	83
Pecan halves, 8	100
Pretzel, soft, plain, ½	95
Prune juice, ½ cup	91
Pudding, prepared from mix, no-fat, no-sugar, ½ cup	70–100
Snack cake, Tastykake, 1 chocolate	90
Snack mix, Chex, ½ cup	100
Soup, cream of potato, 1 cup	73
Soup, cream of shrimp, 1 cup	90
Soup, egg drop, 1 cup	73
Sugar wafers, 2 Keebler	75
Waffle, 1 frozen, spread with 2 tsp apple butter	130
Walnut halves, 7	90
Yogurt, fat-free frozen, ½ cup	95

70 Foods That Are Good or High Sources of Fiber

If you think of fiber as the digestive equivalent of the Roto-Rooter man, stop that thought. Replace that unpleasant visualization with this one: you, only slimmer and healthier, munching on a bowlful of fresh berries. Or a slice of sunny mango. Or a plate of nutty-tasting whole wheat pasta.

Fiber is one of the most potent weapons in your weight-loss arsenal. The more of it you eat—and experts recommend 25 to 35 grams of dietary fiber per day—the more likely you are to lose unwanted pounds. Most high-fiber foods are low in fat and calories, so if you eat lots of them, you'll likely eat fewer calories and less fat. Plus, study after study has found that a fiber-rich diet protects you against all sorts of debilitating diseases, from diabetes to heart disease.

This list can help you meet your daily fiber quota.

Good Fiber Sources

The following foods supply more than 2.5 grams but less than 5 grams of fiber per serving.

Food	Portion	Fiber (g)
Beans and Peas		
Peas, green, boiled	½ cup	3.7–4.4
Soybeans, green, boiled	½ cup	3.8
Cereals		
General Mills Multi-Bran Chex	1 oz	3.7
Kellogg's Cracklin' Oat Bran	1 oz	3.3
Post Fruit & Fibre	1 oz	2.8–3.7

Food	Portion	Fiber (g)
Post Grape-Nuts	1 oz	2.8
Post Original Shredded Wheat, spoon-size	1 oz	2.9
Post Raisin Bran	1 oz	3.8–4.0
Fruit		
Apple, raw with peel	1 medium	3.7
Apricots, dried	10 halves	3.0
Avocado, sliced	½ cup	3.7
Banana	1 medium	2.8
Blackberries, fresh	½ cup	3.8
Cranberries, dried, sweetened	¼ cup	2.5–3.0
Dates, chopped, pitted	¼ cup	3.4
Figs, fresh	2	3.2
Mango, fresh	1 whole	3.7
Orange	1 medium	3.0
Peaches, dried	¼ cup	3.3–4.9
Pear, dried	¼ cup	3.4–4.1
Pear, fresh	1 medium	4.4
Raisins, seedless	½ cup	2.8–3.3
Raspberries, fresh	½ cup	4.2
Nuts and Seeds		
Flaxseed	1 Tbsp	3.3
Sunflower seeds, dry-roasted	1 oz	3.1
Walnuts, black or English	½ cup	3.1–4.0
Vegetables		
Broccoli, frozen, cooked	½ cup	2.8
Brussels sprouts, frozen, cooked	½ cup	3.2
Carrots, frozen, cooked	½ cup	2.6
Greens, turnip or chicory, cooked	½ cup	2.5–3.6
Okra, frozen, cooked	½ cup	2.6

Food	Portion	Fiber (g)
Vegetables *(cont.)*		
Parsnips, boiled, sliced	½ cup	3.1–3.2
Portobello mushroom, raw	1 whole	3.0
Potato, baked	1 long	4.8
Pumpkin, canned	½ cup	3.5
Spinach, frozen, steamed or boiled	½ cup	2.6–2.8
Squash, hubbard or butternut, baked, mashed	½ cup	3.0
Sweet potato, baked	1 medium	3.4

Excellent Fiber Sources

These foods provide more than 5 grams of fiber per serving.

Food	Portion	Fiber (g)
Beans and Peas		
Chickpeas, cooked	½ cup	6.2
Cowpeas or black-eyed peas, cooked	½ cup	5.6
Great Northern beans, cooked	½ cup	6.2
Kidney beans, cooked	½ cup	5.6
Lentils, cooked	½ cup	7.8
Lima beans, cooked	½ cup	6.6
Navy beans, cooked	½ cup	5.8
Pinto beans, cooked	½ cup	7.4
Soybeans, dry-roasted	½ cup	7.0
Soybeans, mature, boiled	½ cup	5.0
Split peas, boiled	½ cup	8.1
White beans, cooked	½ cup	9.4
Cereals		
General Mills Fiber One	1 oz	13.3
Kellogg's All-Bran	1 oz	9.1

Food	Portion	Fiber (g)
Kellogg's All-Bran Bran Buds	1 oz	11.2
Post Bran Flakes	1 oz	5.5
Post 100% Bran	1 oz	8.1
Fruit		
Avocado, pureed/mashed	½ cup	5.6
Figs, dried	¼ cup	6.0
Papaya, fresh	½ cup	5.5
Prunes, uncooked	10	6.0
Raspberries, frozen	½ cup	5.5
Grains		
Barley, cooked	½ cup	6.8
Nuts		
Almonds, whole, dry-roasted, no added salt	½ cup	8.1
Macadamia nuts, dry-roasted, no added salt	½ cup	5.3
Peanuts, dry-roasted, no added salt	½ cup	5.8
Pistachio nuts, dry-roasted, no added salt	½ cup	6.5
Vegetables		
Artichoke, globe, cooked	1	6.5–6.9
Squash, acorn, baked, mashed	½ cup	5.0
Whole wheat products		
Bagel	1 small	5.4
Soft pretzel	1	8.0
Spaghetti, cooked	1 cup	6.3

About the Authors

Cathy Nonas, M.S., R.D., C.D.E., is director of the VanItallie Center for Nutrition and Weight Management, an arm of the New York Obesity Research Center at St. Luke's–Roosevelt Hospital Center in New York City. The Obesity Research Center is one of four federally funded centers for investigating the causes and treatment of obesity in the United States.

Julia VanTine is a health journalist whose most recent books include *Maximum Food Power for Women* and *Energy for Everything: Rejuvenation for the Mind, Body, and Soul.*

Index

Underscored page references indicate boxed text and tables.

Activity. *See also* Exercise
  assessing, with Eating Assessment
    Test, 48–50
  evaluation of, 75–76
  measuring level of, 113
  move tools for, 125–34
  personal story about, <u>122</u>
  for preventing overeating, 121–24
Alcohol
  food tools for handling, 101
  overeating from, 104
  tools for handling, 58–59
American Paradox, 3
Anchovy paste, in hors d'oeuvres,
  <u>275</u>
Angel food cake, serving suggestions
  for, <u>281</u>
Anger
  as Danger Zone, 160
  recipes for overcoming, 241–47
  overeating from, mood tools for
    handling, 60, 120–21
Apple cider
  Hot Mulled Apple-Cranberry Punch,
    279
Apples
  Charoset, 282
  Cranberry-Apple Cobbler, 294
  New-Wave Streusel Apples, 255
  Pitas Stuffed with Chicken-Apple
    Salad, 264
Apricot nectar
  Hot Mulled Cranberry-Apricot Punch,
    279
  Oven-Crisped French Toast with
    Apricot Sauce, 328

Apricots
  Fresh Fruit Tart with Olive Oil Crust,
    272–73
Artichoke hearts, for hors d'oeuvres, <u>275</u>
Arugula
  Spring Greens and Strawberries with
    Poppy Seed Dressing, 284
Attitude adjustments, as mood tool, 106

Baby
  eating profile of, 39
  tips for helping, 61–62
Bananas
  Banana-Chocolate Shake, 322
  Banana Ice Cream with Silky
    Chocolate Sauce, 325
  Grilled Peanut Butter and Banana
    Sandwich, 244
  Strawberries with Creamy Banana
    Sauce, 254
Barbecue sauce
  Barbecued Popcorn, 247
Barhopping
  behavior tools for handling, 142–43
  food tools for handling, 101–2
Barley
  Barley-Corn Pilaf with Jack Cheese,
    238–39
  Beef and Mushroom Barley, 316
Basil
  Herbed Yogurt Cheese Dip, 242
  Mixed Herb Pesto, 308
  Pesto, 308
  Poached Salmon with Toasted Bread
    Crumbs and Basil, 234

Fish. *See also* Shellfish
Bouillabaisse, 298
Cioppino, 299
Mexican Tuna Cobb Salad, 260–61
Pasta Shells in Broth with Tuna, White Beans, and Spinach, 239
Poached Salmon with Toasted Bread Crumbs and Basil, 234
smoked salmon, for hors d'oeuvres, 274–75
Tuna and Zucchini Melts, 265
Fitness level, evaluating, in weight-loss maintenance, 222
500-calorie meals, 339
sample menus for, 342–44
Food diary
analyzing, 214–15
benefits of, 204–5, 206–8
detecting eating motive from, 212–15
detecting eating patterns from, 206–7
effectiveness of, 23
functions of, 22–23, 32, 34
how to keep, 26, 205, 208–9
as mood tool, 105
personal stories about, 132, 152–53, 203–4, 213, 218
for recording bites, tastes, and nibbles, 53–54, 94
types of, 34, 210–11
for weight-loss maintenance, 46, 221
Food policies, personal stories about, 12–13, 64
Food pushers, as Danger Zone, 172
Food shopping, behavior tools for, 151
Food tools, 28
as strategy for
barhopping, buffets, and cocktail parties, 101–2
bread cravings, 82–83
breakfast, 83–84
calorie counting, 84–86
calorie cutting, 86–88
chocolate cravings, 97–99
fat battling, 88–89
hunger blocking, 95–97

increasing fruit and vegetable intake, 89–92
night eating, 99–100
restaurant meals, 102–4
10, to live by, 92–95
Fourth of July recipes, 266–73
French fries
Crab-Boil Oven Fries, 334
Oven Fries, 334
Southwest Oven Fries, 334
Spicy Oven Fries, 334
French Paradox, 3
French-style dishes
Bouillabaisse, 298
French toast
Oven-Crisped French Toast with Apricot Sauce, 328
Fruit juice
avoiding alcoholic drinks with, 101
cutting calories from, 88
Fruits
Banana-Chocolate Shake, 322
Banana Ice Cream with Silky Chocolate Sauce, 325
Charoset, 282
Cherry-Peach Crisp, 270
Chocolate Crêpes with Berries, 319
Coconut Fool, 271
Cranberry-Apple Cobbler, 294
Cranberry-Peach Compote, 256
as dessert, 104
Fresh Fruit Tart with Olive Oil Crust, 272–73
Grilled Peanut Butter and Banana Sandwich, 244
Hot Mulled Apple-Cranberry Punch, 279
Hot Mulled Cranberry-Apricot Punch, 279
Hot Mulled Cranberry-Pear Punch, 279
increasing intake of, 90–91
New-Wave Streusel Apples, 255
Orange-Sauced Crêpes, 326–27
Pear and Smoked Turkey Salad, 259
Pitas Stuffed with Chicken-Apple Salad, 264

Pedometer, for tracking workouts, 126, 134

Peppers, bell
  Broiled Vegetable Kebabs, 269
  Focaccia Bread with Marinated Vegetables, 311
  Grilled Vegetable Sandwich, 262
  Rosemary Roasted Vegetables, 257
  Vegetable Pizza with Goat Cheese, 245
  Vegetables on the Grill, 261
Perfectionism in dieting, FATitude vs. FITitude about, 16–18
Perfectionist, as Inner Saboteur, 43–44
  tips for helping, 70–71
Personal stories
  on using tools, <u>12–13</u>, <u>22–23</u>, <u>46–47</u>, <u>64–65</u>, <u>90–91</u>, <u>122–23</u>, <u>132–33</u>, <u>152–53</u>, <u>180</u>, 203–4, <u>212–13</u>, <u>218–19</u>, <u>224</u>
  on weight-loss maintenance, 216–17
Personal trainers, 131, 134
Pesto, 308
  Mixed Herb Pesto, 308
Pierogies, mini-, as hors d'oeuvres, <u>274</u>
Pies
  Ricotta, Feta, and Spinach Pie, 258
  Turkey Pot Pie with Buttermilk Biscuit Crust, 249
Pilaf
  Barley-Corn Pilaf with Jack Cheese, 238–39
Pineapple
  Tropical Fruit Trifle Parfaits, 273
Pitas
  Greek Skillet Dinner in a Pita, 314–15
  Italian Nachos, 311
  Pitas Stuffed with Chicken-Apple Salad, 264
Pizza
  Greengrocer's Pizza, 335
  Homemade Pizza in a Flash, 235
  Vegetable Pizza with Goat Cheese, 245
Plateau, as Danger Zone, 179
Popcorn
  Barbecued Popcorn, 247
  Chili-Cheese Popcorn, 247

Poppy seeds
  Spring Greens and Strawberries with Poppy Seed Dressing, 284
Popsicles
  Chocolate Frozen Yogurt Pops, 323
Pork
  Glazed Roast Pork Tenderloin, 280
  Pork and Vegetable Stew with Cornmeal Dumplings, 300–301
  Pork Chops with Mexican Peanut Sauce, 237
  smoked ham, for hors d'oeuvres, <u>275</u>
Portions
  controlling
    as behavior tool, 140–42
    personal story about, <u>153</u>
    in restaurants, 103–4, 144
  estimating size of, 93
  promoting obesity, 4
Positive changes, tallying, as mood tool, 112–14
Potatoes
  Baked Potatoes with Chive and Cheese Topping, 292–93
  Baked Vegetable Latkes, 317
  Chicken Roasted with Winter Vegetables, 303
  Crab-Boil Oven Fries, 334
  Creamy Potato Salad, 268
  Light 'n' Lean Nachos, 242–43
  Mashed Potatoes, 248
  for night snack, 99
  omitting, from diet, 85–86
  Oven Fries, 334
  Potato Chips, 241
  Potatoes Stuffed with Turkey Ham, 240
  Southwest Oven Fries, 334
  Spicy Oven Fries, 334
  Whipped Carrots and Potatoes, 291
Pot pie
  Turkey Pot Pie with Buttermilk Biscuit Crust, 249
Pot roast
  Old-Fashioned Pot Roast, 289
Poultry. *See* Chicken; Turkey

Pregnancy weight gain, as Danger Zone, 196
Premenstrual cravings, food tools for controlling, 98–99
Protein
  diets high in, <u>27</u>
  for suppressing appetite, 138
Pudding
  Easy Chocolate Pudding, 322–23
Punch
  Hot Mulled Apple-Cranberry Punch, 279
  Hot Mulled Cranberry-Apricot Punch, 279
  Hot Mulled Cranberry-Pear Punch, 279

food tools, 57, 59, 102–4
mood tools, 57, 59
portion control, 103–4, 144
Restrained Eaters
  eating profile of, 40
  tips for helping, 63, 66
Rewards, as mood tool, 107
Rice
  for night snack, 99
  omitting, from diet, 85–86
  Seafood Paella, 331
Rolls
  Sourdough Hard Rolls, 307
Rope jumping, as move tool, 129
Rosemary
  Rosemary Roasted Vegetables, 257

Quality of life, measuring, 113
Quiche
  Quiche Florentine, 253
Quiz, for assessing eating and exercise program, 76–78

Radishes
  Broiled Vegetable Kebabs, 269
Raisins
  Charoset, 282
Raspberries
  Fresh Fruit Tart with Olive Oil Crust, 272–73
Reading, eating while, as Danger Zone, 176
Rebel, as Inner Saboteur, 44
  tips for helping, 71
Resistance training. See Weight training
Restaurant dining
  handling, with
    behavior tools, 57, 59, 144–45
    external controls, 56

Saboteur, Inner, Eating Assessment Test
  for confronting, 42–45
  evaluation of, 69–72
Salads
  Creamy Potato Salad, 268
  crunchy topper for, 87
  Mexican Tuna Cobb Salad, 260–61
  Pear and Smoked Turkey Salad, 259
  Pitas Stuffed with Chicken-Apple Salad, 264
  for preventing night eating, 99
  Serendipitous Spinach Salad, 293
  Spring Greens and Strawberries with Poppy Seed Dressing, 284
  Zesty Cantaloupe Salad, 266
Salmon
  Poached Salmon with Toasted Bread Crumbs and Basil, 234
  smoked, for hors d'oeuvres, <u>274–75</u>
Salsa
  Fresh Tomato Salsa with Homemade Tortilla Chips, 243
  Spinach Turkey Burgers with Corn Salsa, 267
  uses for, 87

Work(ing) *(cont.)*
at home, as Danger Zone, 170
recipes for, 257–65
Workout, eating after, as Danger Zone, 167

Yogurt
Chocolate Frozen Yogurt Pops, 323
Herbed Yogurt Cheese Dip, 242
Hot-Fudge Sundaes, 254

Zucchini
Baked Vegetable Latkes, 317
Rosemary Roasted Vegetables, 257
Tuna and Zucchini Melts, 265
Vegetables on the Grill, 261
Zucchini in Fresh Tomato Sauce, 292
Zuccotto, 312

Conversion Chart

These equivalents have been slightly rounded to make measuring easier.

Volume Measurements

U.S.	Imperial	Metric
¼ tsp	–	1 ml
½ tsp	–	2 ml
1 tsp	–	5 ml
1 Tbsp	–	15 ml
2 Tbsp (1 oz)	1 fl oz	30 ml
¼ cup (2 oz)	2 fl oz	60 ml
⅓ cup (3 oz)	3 fl oz	80 ml
½ cup (4 oz)	4 fl oz	120 ml
⅔ cup (5 oz)	5 fl oz	160 ml
¾ cup (6 oz)	6 fl oz	180 ml
1 cup (8 oz)	8 fl oz	240 ml

Weight Measurements

U.S.	Metric
1 oz	30 g
2 oz	60 g
4 oz (¼ lb)	115 g
5 oz (⅓ lb)	145 g
6 oz	170 g
7 oz	200 g
8 oz (½ lb)	230 g
10 oz	285 g
12 oz (¾ lb)	340 g
14 oz	400 g
16 oz (1 lb)	455 g
2.2 lb	1 kg

Length Measurements

U.S.	Metric
¼"	0.6 cm
½"	1.25 cm
1"	2.5 cm
2"	5 cm
4"	11 cm
6"	15 cm
8"	20 cm
10"	25 cm
12" (1')	30 cm

Pan Sizes

U.S.	Metric
8" cake pan	20 × 4 cm sandwich or cake tin
9" cake pan	23 × 3.5 cm sandwich or cake tin
11" × 7" baking pan	28 × 18 cm baking tin
13" × 9" baking pan	32.5 × 23 cm baking tin
15" × 10" baking pan	38 × 25.5 cm baking tin (Swiss roll tin)
1½ qt baking dish	1.5 liter baking dish
2 qt baking dish	2 liter baking dish
2 qt rectangular baking dish	30 × 19 cm baking dish
9" pie plate	22 × 4 or 23 × 4 cm pie plate
7" or 8" springform pan	18 or 20 cm springform or loose-bottom cake tin
9" × 5" loaf pan	23 × 13 cm or 2 lb narrow loaf tin or pâté tin

Temperatures

Fahrenheit	Centigrade	Gas
140°	60°	–
160°	70°	–
180°	80°	–
225°	105°	¼
250°	120°	½
275°	135°	1
300°	150°	2
325°	160°	3
350°	180°	4
375°	190°	5
400°	200°	6
425°	220°	7
450°	230°	8
475°	245°	9
500°	260°	–